Preventive Female Sex Factors Against The Development of Chronic Liver Disease

Edited By

Ichiro Shimizu

Department of Gastroenterology,
Seirei Yokohama Hospital,
Kanagawa, Japan

CONTENTS

FOREWORD

The era of individualized medicine has arrived in the field of hepatology. Medicine based on genetic polymorphisms is a growing trend, especially for patients with chronic liver diseases arising from infection with hepatitis C virus (HCV), an endemic disease in Japan. In August 2009, single nucleotide polymorphisms (SNPs) of IL-28B, also known as interferon-λ, were shown to be an important host factor affecting the efficacy of ribavirin and pegylated interferon therapy in patients with chronic hepatitis C. As of July 2010, the Japanese Ministry of Health, Welfare, and Labor has allowed the use of these SNPs for advanced medical care to predict the therapeutic efficacy of given treatments in individual patients. Also in 2010, SNPs of the inosine triphosphatase (ITPA) gene were found to be a host factor determining the extent of hemolytic anemia caused by ribavirin, and it seems that genetic factors contributing to the development of other adverse effects, such as neutrocytopenia, thrombocytopenia and interstitial pneumonia, are likely to be identified in the near future. A genome-wide association study (GWAS) of SNPS will enable hepatologists to achieve such notable progresses, possibly clarifying the mechanisms involved in persistent infections of HCV.

While individualized medicine is a recent trend in hepatology, it has also been part of traditional approaches in ancient medicine traditions arising in Asian countries, including Japan. More than ten centuries ago in Europe, Christian clergies performed therapeutic procedures for various diseases based on their religious dogma. Phlebitis was performed for all patients, regardless of the type of disease and even among those afflicted with plague, according to the theory established by Galenus in Greece during the mid-second century AD. Such medical practices were performed in a uniform manner based on the hypothesis that all diseases developed as a result of imbalances among the four humors (blood, yellow bile, black bile, and phlegm) that had been described by Hippocrates during the fifth century BC. In contrast, in medieval Japan, traditional medicine was established by Buddhist priests based on superstitious divination as well as their religious world views. They used various types of herbs for therapeutic procedures, and different mixtures of numerous herbs were given to patients even if they had the same disease depending on their facial color and the size and strength of the pulse of each patient. These therapeutic approaches have evolved into modern Kanpo-medicine, a traditional form of individualized medicine in Japan.

Although the condition of the pulse and genomic polymorphisms are useful parameters in algorithms for individualized treatment in Kanpo-medicine and recent hepatology, respectively, all physicians would likely agree that the age and sex of the patients are the most important factors in the individualized treatment of various diseases. In patients with a persistent HCV infection, for example, liver fibrosis progresses more rapidly in men than in women. Thus, women with HCV infection generally tend to develop hepatocellular carcinoma later in life than men. Also, the efficacy of ribavirin and pegylated interferon therapy is well known to be superior in women than in men among patients with chronic hepatitis C in Europe and the United States, while the therapeutic efficacy has been shown to be superior in male patients than in female patients in Japan. Moreover, autoimmune hepatitis and primary biliary cirrhosis are frequent diseases among elderly women, but are rare in men of any age. Although the frequency of non-alcoholic fatty liver diseases is greater in men than in women in Japan, the incidence of non-alcoholic fatty liver diseases increases according to age only in women. These fundamental observations in clinical hepatology have prompted us to recognize that sex, as well as age, is an essential factor for establishing algorithms to perform individualized medicine in patients with liver diseases. All of these topics are discussed in the chapter of this eBook entitled, "Preventive Female Sex Factors against the Development of Chronic Liver Disease".

This distinguished and challenging eBook was edited by Dr. Ichiro Shimizu, a pioneer in sex- and/or gender-specific medicine, especially for liver diseases, in Japan. Ten excellent articles written by specialists in various fields of hepatology, such as viral hepatitis, autoimmune liver diseases, alcoholic and non-alcoholic fatty liver disease, and hepatocellular carcinoma, are presented in this eBook. Readers of this eBook will be able to obtain consensus information regarding sex differences in liver diseases. I believe that this eBook will be useful for all researchers and clinicians working in the field of hepatology, serving as a bible for sex- and/or gender-specific medicine, and may contribute to progress in individualized medicine regardless of the therapeutic approach: either modern medicine focusing on genetic polymorphisms or Kanpo-medicine using various herbs.

Satoshi Mochida
Saitama Medical University
Saitama, Japan

PREFACE

Until the last decade, it seemed that women and men were essentially identical except for the differences in their reproductive function. Everywhere, however, researchers look for differences between the sexes, and they find them. Sex does really matter. One of the most compelling reasons for understanding the biological differences is that there are striking differences in human disease. The best-studied differences between the sexes are in the reproductive systems. Much less study has been done on sex differences in non-reproductive areas of biology. It should be noted that liver cancer is undeniably predominant in men and postmenopausal women.

Chronic hepatitis C virus and hepatitis B virus infections are recognized as a major causative factor of cirrhosis and liver cancer. Obesity is also associated with increased incidence rates for cirrhosis and liver cancer. In general, men have a greater risk of exposure to hepatitis viruses, a greater opportunity for drinking, and a higher preponderance of nutritional and exercise-related problems such as obesity. Although it has been speculated that such gender-specific lifestyles and social environments might contribute to the predominant incidence of liver cancer in men, few studies have been done on the biological mechanisms underlying the sex-associated differences observed in chronic liver disease. A characteristic feature of chronic hepatitis C and B, alcoholic liver disease and non-alcoholic fatty liver disease is fatty liver, or hepatic steatosis. Central obesity (android pattern) is a predictor of hepatic steatosis. Hepatic steatosis leads to an increase in lipid peroxidation in hepatocytes, which, in turn, activates hepatic stellate cells (HSCs). HSCs are located in close contact with hepatocytes, and are the primary target cells for inflammatory and oxidative stimuli in the injured liver. Activated HSCs are responsible for much of the collagen synthesis during fibrosis development to the end-stage cirrhosis. Cirrhosis is an important host-related risk factor for liver cancer. Chronic hepatitis C and B appear to progress more rapidly in males than in females. Women have lower hepatic iron stores before menopause, and their production of proinflammatory cytokines, such as tumor necrosis factor-α and interleukin-6, increases after menopause as a result of the decline in ovarian function. Iron is essential for life, but is toxic in excess, because it produces reactive oxygen species (ROS) that react readily with lipids and DNA, leading to cell death and DNA mutagenesis. In addition, hepatic steatosis and central obesity are observed in growth hormone deficiency in adults. Growth hormone secretion is greater in women and is stimulated by estrogen. Estrogen is a potent endogenous antioxidant and suppresses hepatic fibrosis. Estrogen also attenuates hepatocyte death and HSC activation by inhibiting the ROS generation. These lines of evidence suggest that the greater progression of hepatic fibrosis and liver cancer in men and postmenopausal women may be due, at least in part, to lower secretions of estrogen and growth hormone, higher hepatic iron stores and increased immune responses.

Using gender and sex as a unique prism through which to observe and better understand normal function and the experience of disease is one of the most important new ideas in medicine. This e-Book constitutes a collection of selected clinical and scientific topics in conjunction with the sex-associated differences of the liver disease. After considering the data and examples presented in the e-Book, anyone will be able to use new opportunities to obtain a better understanding of the sex-associated differences of chronic liver disease. Some of these differences can be explained by what we now know. Some are unexplained and point to important questions for future study. Being female or male is an important basic human variable that affects health and liver disease throughout the life span. A better understanding of the biological mechanisms underlying the differences in chronic liver disease between the sexes would provide valuable information to design care of health and liver disease more effectively for individuals, both females and males.

Ichiro Shimizu,
Department of Gastroenterology,
Seirei Yokohama Hospital,
Kanagawa, Japan

CONTRIBUTORS

Chiaki Sagara	Support Center for Medical Sciences, Seirei Yokohama Hospital, 215 Iwai-cho, Hodogaya-ku, Kanagawa 240-8521, Japan
Claudio Puoti	Professor of Department of Internal Medicine and Liver Unit, Marino Hospital, Viale XXIV Maggio, 00047 Marino, Roma, Italy
Hayato Nakagawa	Department of Gastroenterology, University of Tokyo, 7-3-1 Hongo, Bunkyo-ku, Tokyo 113-8655, Japan
Ichiro Shimizu	A.G.A.F., Department of Gastroenterology, Seirei Yokohama Hospital, 215 Iwai-cho, Hodogaya-ku, Kanagawa 240-8521, Japan
Kittiyod Poovorawan	Department of Medicine, Faculty of Medicine, Chulalongkorn University, Bangkok 10330, Thailand
Nozomi Suzuki	Support Center for Medical Sciences, Seirei Yokohama Hospital, 215 Iwai-cho, Hodogaya-ku, Kanagawa 240-8521, Japan
Pisit Tangkijvanich	Associate Professor of Department of Biochemistry, Faculty of Medicine, Chulalongkorn University, Bangkok 10330, Thailand
Satoshi Mochida	Professor & Chairman, Department of Gastroenterology & Hepatology, Faculty of Medicine, Saitama Medical University, 38 Morohongo, Moroyama-machi, Iruma-gun, Saitama 350-0495, Japan
Sumiko Nagoshi	Professor of Department of Gastroenterology & Hepatology, Faculty of Medicine, Saitama Medical University, 38 Morohongo, Moroyama-machi, Iruma-gun, Saitama 350-0495, Japan
Takato Ueno	Professor of Research Center for Innovative Cancer Therapy, Kurume University, 67 Asahi-machi, Kurume 830–0011, Japan
Tomomi Matsumoto	Support Center for Medical Sciences, Seirei Yokohama Hospital, 215 Iwai-cho, Hodogaya-ku, Kanagawa 240-8521, Japan
Tsutoshi Asaki	Department of Gastroenterology, Seirei Yokohama Hospital, 215 Iwai-cho, Hodogaya-ku, Kanagawa 240-8521, Japan
Yong Poovorawan	Professor of Center of Excellence in Clinical Virology, Faculty of Medicine, Chulalongkorn University, Bangkok 10330, Thailand
Yoshiki Katakura	Department of Gastroenterology, Seirei Yokohama Hospital, 215 Iwai-cho, Hodogaya-ku, Kanagawa 240-8521, Japan
Yosho Fukita	Department of Gastroenterology, Seirei Yokohama Hospital, 215 Iwai-cho, Hodogaya-ku, Kanagawa 240-8521, Japan
Yui Koizumi	Support Center for Medical Sciences, Seirei Yokohama Hospital, 215 Iwai-cho, Hodogaya-ku, Kanagawa 240-8521, Japan

CHAPTER 1

Chronic Liver Diseases Develop More Slowly in Females Than Males

Ichiro Shimizu[1*], **Tomomi Matsumoto**[2], **Nozomi Suzuki**[2], **Chiaki Sagara**[2], **Yui Koizumi**[2], **Tsutoshi Asaki**[1], **Yoshiki Katakura**[1] and **Yosho Fukita**[1]

[1]*Department of Gastroenterology and* [2]*Support Center for Medical Sciences, Seirei Yokohama Hospital, 215 Iwai-cho, Hodogaya-ku, Kanagawa 240-8521, Japan*

Abstract: More than 350 million and 170 million people worldwide are persistently infected with hepatitis B virus (HBV) and hepatitis C virus (HCV), respectively. Chronic HBV infection is the most common cause of cirrhosis and hepatocellular carcinoma (HCC) in the world, while HCV infection is the main cause of cirrhosis and HCC in Japan, Europe, and the United States. Cirrhosis and HCC are predominantly diseases which tend to occur in men and postmenopausal women. Differences in the social environment and the lifestyles of women and men may be involved in the basic mechanisms underlying the sex-associated differences in progression of HCV and HBV infection. In general, males have a greater risk of exposure to hepatitis viruses as well as a greater opportunity for drinking. Environmental factors may result in a higher preponderance of nutritional and exercise-associated problems in males. Females, particularly before menopause, could produce antibodies against HBV surface antigen and e antigen at a higher frequency than males among HBV carriers. The progression time from chronic hepatitis C to cirrhosis is found to be longer in females than in males. Male sex, older age ($\geq$50 years) and cirrhosis are important host-related risk factors for the development of HCC. Therefore, cases of female sex and under 50 years old, namely "premenopausal women" are least vulnerable to HCC.

Keywords: Sex-associated difference, male predominance, menopause, sex hormone, male-to-female ratio, HBV, HCV, hepatocellular carcinoma, cirrhosis, environment, lifestyle, drinking, slow progression.

1. INTRODUCTION

Hepatitis C virus (HCV) infections are more common than hepatitis B virus (HBV) infections in Japan and Western countries, and are recognized as a major causative factor of chronic hepatitis, cirrhosis, and hepatocellular carcinoma (HCC). Cirrhosis is a greatest risk factor for HCC [1,2]. Among patients with cirrhosis and HCC, the male: female ratio is in the range of 2.3:1 to 2.6:1 [3-5].

Differences in social environment and lifestyle of men and women may be involved in the basic mechanisms underlying the sex-associated differences of these chronic liver diseases. In general, there are more men with an opportunity to come into contact with a hepatitis virus and an opportunity for drinking [6-9]. Environmental features of male gender may lead to a greater preponderance for nutritional and exercise problem for men [10-12]. However, it should be noted that some mechanisms of the sex-associated differences may be based on biological factors, including estrogen of female sex hormones rather than on gender differences in social environment and lifestyle. The present chapter summarizes our current knowledge of the sex-associated clinical observations as it relates to the progression of chronic liver disease.

2. HCV AND HBV INFECTIONS IN THE WORLD

More than 350 million and 170 million people worldwide are persistently infected with HBV [13] and HCV [14], respectively. Chronic HBV infection is the most common cause of cirrhosis and HCC in the world. The prevalence of chronic HBV infection is widely variable in different parts of the world [15] (Fig. **1**). Low prevalence areas include North America, Southern South America, Northern and Western Europe, and Australia and New Zealand. Intermediate prevalence rates occur in most areas surrounding the Amazon

*Address correspondence to Ichiro Shimizu:** Department of Gastroenterology, Seirei Yokohama Hospital, 215 Iwai-cho, Hodogaya-ku, Yokohama, Kanagawa 240-8521, Japan; Tel: +81-45-715-3111; Fax: +81-45-715-3387; E-mail: ichiro.shimizu@showaclinic.jp

River basin, Southern and Eastern Europe, Russian Federation, South-Central Asia, and Japan. High prevalence areas include the interior Amazon River basin, all of Africa except for Mediterranean countries, South-Eastern Asia, China, and Korea. The mode of transmission of HBV varies and is related to the prevalence of the infection in an area of the world. In high prevalence areas, the most common mode of transmission tends to be mother-to-child (perinatal) infection. In areas with an intermediate prevalence of HBV, the primary mode of transmission appears to be child-to-child (horizontal) transmission, particularly in early childhood [16]. In lower prevalence areas, such as in the United States, Northern, Western and Southern Europe, and Australia, acquisition of HBV infection at birth or during childhood is rare, and the most common mode of transmission of HBV is unprotected sexual intercourse and injection drug use in young adults [17]. Importantly, infection with HBV can be prevented by the highly effective recombinant vaccination that is available. If global vaccination practices could be implemented, HBV could be controlled and virtually eradicated.

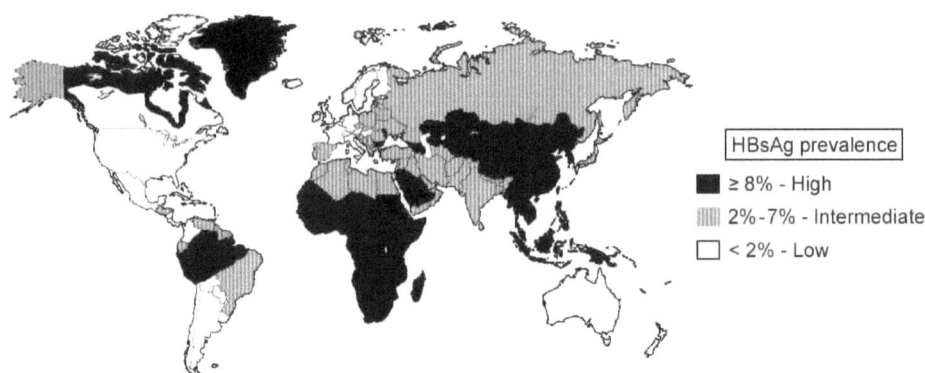

Fig. 1. Geographic distribution of HBV infection [15]. Positivity for HBV surface antigen (HBsAg) means HBV infection.

HCV infection is endemic in most parts of the world. HCV infection is the main cause of the end-stage cirrhosis and HCC in the United States, Europe, and Japan. The burden of disease is expected to increase in the next decade. HCV is currently an important public health issue worldwide. Similar to HBV, geographic differences in endemicity of HCV infection can be described based on regional prevalences; high (prevalence rate ≥3%), moderate (prevalence rate 2%-2.9%), low (prevalence rate 1.0%-1.9%), and very low (prevalence rate <1.0%) [17]. However, the regions corresponding to these prevalences are different for HCV than for HBV. Highest prevalence of HCV infection has been reported from Northern Africa (particularly Egypt), moderate prevalence from Eastern Europe and most of Asia, low prevalence from Northern and South America, Western Europe and Australia, and very low prevalence from Northern Europe and the United Kingdom.

Table 1. Exposures known to be associated with HCV infection

Transfusion, transplant from HCV-infected donors
Unsafe therapeutic (iatrogenic) injections
Injection drug use
Tattoos
Occupational exposure to HCV-infected blood (mostly contaminated needle sticks)
Sex with HCV-infected partner (multiple sex partners)
Birth to HCV-infected mother

It only became possible to test for HCV after the genomic sequence of the virus was identified in 1989. Prior to this time HCV was clinically recognized as a form of hepatitis commonly occurring after blood transfusions. Substantial differences in the endemicity of HCV infection are related to frequency and extent to which various risk factors contributed to transmission. Routes by which individuals may have been exposed to HCV include receiving of blood products or transplanted solid organs, transfusion of clotting factors, unsafe therapeutic injections, intravenous drug use, or tattoos (Table 1). Because HCV has been molecularly characterized, screening the blood supply and potential organ donors is possible and the risk associated with transfusion and transplants has markedly diminished. Illegal injection drug use remains a very common way that people acquire HCV in most developed countries. In many cases, a clear risk factor or exposure is never identified. HCV is not usually transmitted by routine household contact. A few behaviors should be avoided including sharing razors, toothbrushes, and any practices in which the possibility of blood exposure is high. HCV can be transmitted sexually, but this is not a common route. In fact, the risk of sexual transmission appears to be very low in monogamous couples in which one partner is positive for HCV and the other is not. It does appear that as in the case of other sexually transmitted diseases male to female transmission may be more efficient. Sexual practices that may be associated with increased risk of HCV transmission include having multiple partners, other sexually transmitted diseases, sex with trauma, and non-use of condoms. In general, males have a greater risk of exposure to HCV [8,12,18].

If an HBV infection is acquired by the newborn, there is a chance of becoming chronically infected. However, if it is acquired during adulthood, this risk is relatively low (approximately 10% to 20%) [19,20]. Fifteen to 40% of chronically infected people may develop cirrhosis and HCC [21]. The remaining individuals become inactive carriers, otherwise defined as asymptomatic carriers. Asymptomatic carriers show seropositivity for HBsAg with normal liver enzyme ALT levels for 6 months or more. In a meta-analysis of 32 case-control studies conducted in diverse populations and comprising roughly 4500 cases of HCC and 7000 control subjects, the risk for HCC is increased 20-fold in HBV carriers compared with HBV-negative controls (95% confidence interval: 18- to 23-fold) [22]. In contrast, about 80% of adults infected with HCV progress to chronic hepatitis [23]. HCV seems to be associated with HCC in areas with a relatively low prevalence of HBV infection. For example, in the United States, Europe, and Japan, HCV accounts for 47%-55%, 44%-66%, and 75% of HCC cases, respectively [24-26]. In China and Africa, HCV is associated with less than 5% of cases. In the meta-analysis of 32 case-control studies, the HCC risk is increased 24-fold in HCV-infected patients compared with HCV-negative controls (95% confidence interval: 20- to 28-fold) [22].

3. CLINICAL REMISSION OR SLOW PROGRESSION IN FEMALES WITH HBV INFECTION

During the early phase of chronic HBV infection, patients are positive for HBV e antigen (HBeAg), a surrogate marker of active HBV replication. They have frequent acute flares characterized by substantial increases in the blood alanine aminotransferase (ALT) levels as the result of specific, T-lymphocyte-mediated cellular responses to viral antigens and apoptosis of hepatocytes. Some acute flares may be followed by seroconversion from HBeAg to its antibody (anti-HBe) and clinical remission [27,28]. Among HBV carriers, a few progress to cirrhosis and HCC, particularly in elderly male persons [29,30]. Males appear to have more severe disease, with a faster progression to cirrhosis [31]. Positivity for HBeAg is associated with a higher inflammatory activity in the liver and an increased risk of HCC [32]. An analysis of 6,342 asymptomatic carriers of HBV in Japan showed that the rates of positivity for HBeAg and anti-HBe were 16.7% and 53.1% in female donors, and 19.1% and 49.6% in males, respectively [33]. Seroconversion from HBeAg to anti-HBe occurs more frequently in females than in males [34] (Table 2).

Table 2. Favorable virological reactions in female patients with HBV infection as compared with those in males

Higher clearance of HBsAg in females
Higher seroconversion from HBeAg to anti-HBe in females
Higher production of anti-HBs after HBV vaccination in females

Liver injury in chronic hepatitis B is predominantly caused by the cellular immune response to the HBV, and the balance between HBV and the immune response changes over time [35]. Generally, females produce more vigorous cellular and humoral immune reactions [36]. The prevalence of HBsAg is reported to be higher in males than in females throughout the world [37]. In a prospective follow-up study of up to 19 years on HBsAg carriers in Okinawa in Japan, clearance of HBsAg was found more frequently in females (7.8%) than in males (5.8%) [38]. The underlying mechanism by which females seem more likely to develop HBsAg clearance and HBeAg seroconversion remains vague. However, a sex hormone, estradiol, which represents the major estrogen, has been reported to augment an antigen-specific primary antibody response in human peripheral blood mononuclear cells [39]. Thus, female individuals, particularly before menopause, could produce antibodies against HBsAg and HBeAg at a higher frequency than males among HBV carriers.

Eight types (A to H) of the HBV DNA characterization (genotype) are currently recognized. The genotypes show a distinct geographical distribution between and even within regions. Structural and functional differences between genotypes can influence the severity, course and likelihood of complications and HBeAg seroconversion. Patients infected with HBV genotype C is shown to have delayed HBeAg seroconversion, longer periods of viremia, a greater risk of progressive disease, and a correspondingly higher rate of cirrhosis and HCC [40]. Genotypes C and B are prevalent in Asia, whereas genotypes A and D prevail in Western countries. An increasing prevalence of HBeAg-negative chronic hepatitis B has recently been observed in many countries [41,42]. The HBeAg-negative chronic hepatitis B patients are usually males and older than those with HBeAg-positive chronic hepatitis B [42].

Immunization is the most effective way to prevent the transmission of HBV. After appropriate immunization with HBV vaccine, approximately 90% of healthy adults and 95% of infants, children, and adolescents develop a protective blood level of the antibody to HBsAg (anti-HBs). The predictors associated with a non-response to HBV vaccination, however, include male sex, older age, obesity and immunocompromising chronic disease [43]. After an initial vaccination in newborns of Alaska natives with seronegativity for HBsAg and anti-HBs at birth, the mean concentrations of anti-HBs appeared to be higher in females (975 mIU/mL) than in males (722 mIU/mL), but they decreased to 23 mIU/mL for females in comparison to 32 mIU/mL for males 15 years after the first vaccination [44]. In Taiwan, chronic HBsAg carrier rates declined more obviously for females (4.4%) than for males (10.7%) who were born to HBsAg carrier mothers, vaccinated against HBV at birth, and followed up for over 18 years [45].

In a prospective follow-up study on development of 1400 HBsAg-positive Alaska native carriers, the annual incidence of chronic hepatitis and cirrhosis was 158 and 95 per 100,000 for females, and 193 and 107 per 100,000 for males, respectively [46]. In another prospective study from Italy on progression of 25 female and 80 male patients with chronic hepatic B, cirrhosis developed in 2 (8%) in females and 19 (24%) in males during a mean histological follow up of 3.7 years [47]. In this study, the histological diagnosis was made by follow up liver biopsy. In addition, multivariate analysis with patients with chronic HBV infection in France [48] and in Taiwan [31] have showed that independent predictors for cirrhosis include a male sex and an age of older than 50 years. In the United States, male sex and old age are also reported to be the most important factors associated with progression of the disease in chronic hepatitis B [49]. These data show that female sex may be a favorable factor associated with clinical remission or slow progression of HBV carriers.

4. SLOW PROGRESSION FROM CHRONIC HEPATITIS C TO CIRRHOSIS IN FEMALES

An analysis of first-time blood donors in Japan showed that anti-HCV was equally detected in females and males [50]. In the United States, however, male sex is identified as an independent risk factors for HCV seropositivity among 862,398 blood donors (odds ratio, 1.9; 95% confidence interval, 1.8 to 2.1) [51]. A study conducted in Spain, the United Kingdom, France, Switzerland, and Italy showed that male sex was associated with a increased risk of HCV transmission to health care workers after occupational exposure to HCV-infected blood or body fluids (odds ratio, 3.1; 95% confidence interval, 1.0-10.0) [52]. In a report from Egypt, where prevalence rate of HCV is the highest in the world, based on the data of anti-HCV-positive residents, the clearance rate of HCV RNA, in the blood was higher in females (44.6%) than in males (33.7%) [53].

HCV infection is generally slow progressive. Once a person has been exposed to HCV, about 20% of individuals will recover completely while about 80% will go on to develop chronic infection with persistently detectable HCV RNA in the blood. Of this 80% developing chronic infection, approximately

20% to 30% will have severe progression of their liver disease and may develop cirrhosis in 20-30 years and have an increased risk for HCC [23]. About one-third of patients despite detectable HCV RNA in the blood have an asymptomatic disease with persistently normal liver enzyme ALT. In most so called "asymptomatic" carriers of HCV, liver histology shows only mild disease (histologically minimal to mild chronic hepatitis) [54], and levels of HCV RNA in the blood are lower than in those with a raised ALT [55]. However, patients aged over 50 years can be predicated to develop cirrhosis from initially mild disease in half (15-20 years) the time interval estimated for patients aged less than 35 years (time to cirrhosis: 30-40 years or more) [56]. Moreover, in a study from Japan, the intervals between date of blood transfusion and diagnosis of HCC were 29.0 years in 1990, and 36.6 years in 2003 [25]. This estimated incubation period from onset of HCV infection to clinical diagnosis of HCC has also been found in Los Angeles in the United States, where the average interval between blood transfusion and diagnosis of chronic hepatitis as 13.7 years, cirrhosis as 20.6 years, and HCC as 28.3 years [57].

For the sex disparity in the natural history of HCV infection, the progression time from chronic hepatitis C to cirrhosis is found to be longer in females than in males [58-61]. Indeed the progression to cirrhosis is almost 10-fold faster in males irrespective of age [62]. In addition, demographic data from the United States [63], Europe (France and Italy) [54,64], and Japan [65] show that most HCV carriers with persistently normal ALT (asymptomatic carriers) are females, and have a good prognosis with a low risk of progression to cirrhosis (Fig. **2**). These data show that, besides chronic hepatitis B, chronic hepatitis C also appears to progress to cirrhosis more slowly in females than in males. It is noteworthy that the risk of development of HCC in female individuals with chronic hepatitis C in the absence of underlying cirrhosis is quite low.

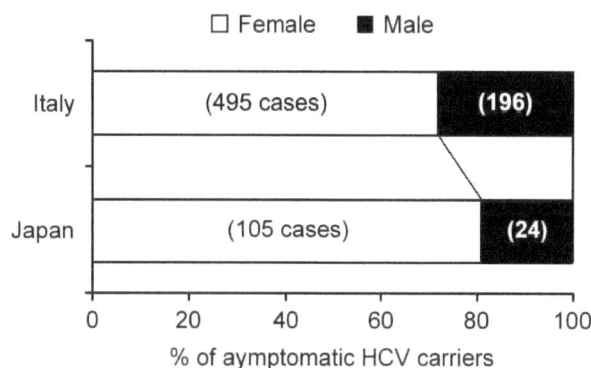

Fig. 2. Female predominance among asymptomatic HCV carriers. Asymptomatic HCV carriers are defined as persistently HCV RNA positive persons with normal blood ALT levels over a 6- to 36-month period. The definitions of "normal" ALT levels are different among studies: < 40 IU/L in Italy [54]; ≤ 30 IU/L in Japan [65].

5. INTERFERON THERAPY FOR CHRONIC HEPATITIS C IN FEMALES

The high frequency of chronicity in HCV infection and evidence of high rates of HCV mutations may be due to either an ineffective immune response or immunological escape by HCV. Chronic HCV infection is a major causative factor for cirrhosis and HCC in the United States, Europe, Australia, and Japan. The initial approved treatment for HCV, interferon-α, has been currently replaced by combination treatment with pegylated interferon-α and ribavirin. Interferon-α appears to have both immunomodulatory and antiviral effects in treating HCV infection. Ribavirin has no antiviral activity as a monotherapy, but it is synergistic with interferons through unknown mechanisms. Pegylated interferon allows for dosing once weekly, whereas non-pegylated short-acting interferon is generally administrated 3 times per week. The goal of treatment with interferon and ribavirin is to achieve a permanent eradication of the virus, or a Sustained Virologic Response (SVR). SVR is defined as the absence of detectable HCV RNA in the blood at the end of treatment and at least 6 months after the cessation of therapy. There are at least six genotypes of HCV RNA (1 to 6). Predictors of a poor response to the treatment include HCV genotypes 1 or 4, high blood levels of HCV RNA, histological evidence of cirrhosis, and male sex (Table **3**). HCV genotype 1 is the most common genotype in the United States, Italy, and Japan.

Table 3. Major risk factors predicting a poor response to interferon-based antiviral therapy in chronic hepatitis C

Virus-related factors	HCV genotypes 1 or 4
	High HCV RNA in the blood
Host-related factors	High histological stage in the liver
	Male sex

Combination therapy with pegylated interferon and ribavirin produces a SVR in approximately 40% to 50% of treated patients with HCV genotype 1 infection [66]. In the United States, the SVR rate to the combination therapy in patients (n=401, median age 43-45 years) with chronic hepatitis C was higher in females than in males [67]. In contrast, in Japanese patients (n=264, median age 54 years) given such combination therapy, the SVR rate showed no sex differences among patients under 50 years of age, and was higher in males than in females among patients aged 50 years and older [68]. Precise estimates are not currently available for the combination of pegylated interferon plus ribavirin, but the discrepancy of the SVR rates among females may be associated with at least the median age difference between treated patient groups. Before 1998 in the initial treatment for chronic hepatitis C, a randomized placebo-controlled trial of short-acting interferon-based antiviral therapy was conducted in Canada, Europe, Israel, and Australia. The SVR rate to short-acting interferon plus ribavirin combination was found to be higher in females than in males [69]. Moreover, short-acting interferon monotherapy achieved a higher SVR rate in females than in males among patients aged younger than 40 years and showed no sex differences among patients aged 40 years and older [70].

During perimenopause from age 40 to 45 years, ovaries start to shut down, and blood gonadotoropin levels frequently reach menopausal levels, even when blood estrogen levels are within the menstrual range [71]. The above data that pre-perimenopausal female patients have a favorable response to interferon-based antiviral therapy, thus, suggest that estrogen levels may be associated with immune responses, which are distinct between females and males.

6. WORLDWIDE INCIDENCE AND SEX RATIOS OF LIVER CANCER

Estimates of the worldwide liver cancer incidence and mortality in the year 2002 are available in the GLOBOCAN series of the International Agency for Research on Cancer [72], which is established in 1965 by the World Health Organization (WHO). According to the WHO, cancer is a leading cause of death worldwide, accounting for 13% of all death. Liver cancer is the third leading cause of cancer mortality (598,000 deaths), exceeded only by cancer of lung and stomach [73]. Liver cancer is a more common cause of death than cancer of colon or breast, and sixth commonly diagnosed cancers (626,000 cases) in the world. Owing to the lack of symptoms in the early stages and the rapid growth rate of tumors, most cases of liver cancer are discovered at an advanced stage, and have the very poor prognosis. Its yearly fatality ratio is approximately 1 (incidence rate very close to mortality rate), indicating that most cases do not survive a year. In Europe, for the period 1990 to 1999 [74], and, in the United States, for the period 1995 to 2000 [75], liver cancer survival rates at the population level showed that the 5-year relative survival rate were 6.5% and 8.3%, respectively. During the last two decades, however, increases of primary liver cancer incidence rates have been reported from the United States [76], Central Europe [77,78], the United Kingdom [79], Australia [80], and Japan [25].

The GLOBOCAN estimates from the year 2002 demonstrate that 184,043 new cases of liver cancer (29% of the total) in females and 442,119 new cases (71% of the total) in males occurred worldwide. This tumor accounted for 5.7% of all new cancers (3.6% among females and 7.6% among males) making it the eighth most common in females, following breast, cervix uteri, colon, lung, stomach, ovary, and corpus uteri cancer, and the fifth most common malignancy in males (following lung, prostate, stomach, and colon cancer) [72]. The commonest primary malignant tumor of the liver in adults is HCC. HCC arises from liver cells (hepatocytes) and accounts for up to 85% of the primary liver cancer cases. Cholangiocarcinoma, another liver cancer, is a relatively rare cancer derived from the intrahepatic bile duct cells; worldwide it accounts for an estimated 15% of liver cancer. Despite a rather wide range in the incidence of liver cancer as a whole, the incidence of cholangiocarcinoma shows rather little variation, with rates in males mainly ranging 0.5-2.0 and a little lower in females [81].

According to the GLOBOCAN 2002 data [72], 82% of liver cancer cases are in developing countries, and 55% are in China alone. The areas of high incidence are Middle (sub-Saharan) Africa and Eastern (China, Taiwan, Korea, and Japan) and South-Eastern Asia. The incidence is low in developed areas (only in Southern Europe is there any substantial risk), South America, and South-Central Asia. Based on the age-adjusted incidence rates of liver cancer registered in different countries in the world, male cases have higher liver cancer rates than female cases in most populations [82]. Age-adjusted incidence rates represent averages per 100,000 using the world population as a standard. Accordingly, the rate is adjusted upward in countries where the average age is low and artificially lowered in countries where the average age is higher; this provides a useful method to more accurately compare average rates between countries. The male-to-female ratio of the age-standardized incidence per 100,000 of liver cancer is 2.7 for the whole world (Fig. 3). Although the sex ratio is similar in less developed countries (2.6) and more developed countries (2.8), it is much greater in the areas of high incidence and less in low incidence areas. It ranges from 1.0 in Central America and to 1.3 in South America, 1.9 in South-Central Asia and North Africa, 2.0 in Northern Europe, 2.1 in Middle Africa, 2.2 in Eastern Europe, 2.3 in Western Asia, 2.5 in Eastern Asia, 2.7 in Western Africa, 2.8 in Eastern Africa, Northern America, and Southern Africa, 2.9 in Southern Europe, 3.2 in South-Eastern Asia and 3.6 in Western Europe [72].

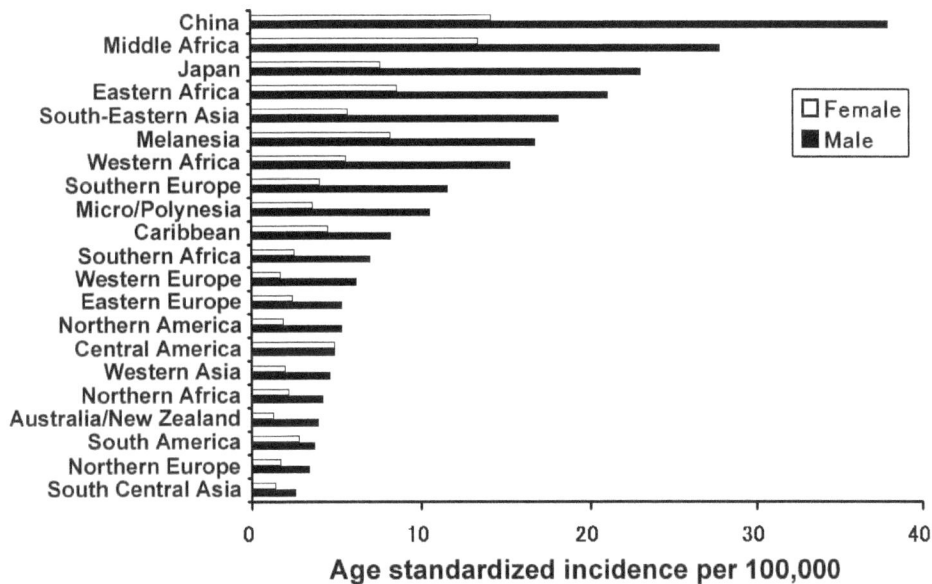

Fig. 3. Age-standardized incidence per 100,000 of liver cancer by sex in different geographic regions worldwide in the year 2002 [72].

In particular, Qidong in the inshore region of the Yangtze River in eastern China has the highest incidence of liver cancer in the world [82]. In Qidong, the age-adjusted incidence rates range from 24.6 to 34.4 for females and from 75.9 to 109.2 for males, and the sex ratios range from 2.9 to 4.0 for the period 1980 to 2002 [83]. The large majority of liver cancer cases occur in patients with chronic infections with either HBV or HCV. Persistent viral infections lead to chronic hepatitis and the end-stage cirrhosis. Overall, 75% to 80% of liver cancer cases are attributable to chronic HBV (50%-55%) and HCV (25%-30%) infections. Thus the reasons for the ratio disparity in different geographic regions in the world may include different environmental and lifestyle factors such as a prevalence of persistent HBV or HCV infection, heavy alcohol intake, and dietary exposure to the carcinogenic toxin aflatoxin produced by molds (Table **4**). Highly aflatoxin-exposed populations are primarily those residing in sub-Saharan Africa and east and southeast Asia.

Table 4. Environmental and lifestyle major risk factors for HCC

HBV infection	Induces chronic hepatitis and cirrhosis
HCV infection	Induces chronic hepatitis and cirrhosis
Heavy alcohol intake	Induces alcoholic cirrhosis and acts as a cofactor in the presence of coexistent infection with HBV and/or HCV
Aflatoxin exposure	Interacts synergistically with HBV infection

For examples, Qidong in China has the highest HCC incidence due to a high prevalence of HBV infection and high levels of aflatoxin. Aflatoxin is found in contaminated foods such as corn and peanuts, and interacts synergistically with HBV infection to amplify the risk of HCC [84]. In Qidong, 84% cases with HCC were seropositive for marker of HBV infection, HBsAg, and 10% were seropositive for HCV infection marker, anti-HCV [85,86]. Because HBV is more prevalence than HCV, the distribution of HBV infection worldwide largely explains the patterns of HCC. The exception is Japan, where chronic infection with HBV is relatively low, but where the generations most at risk of HCC have a relatively high rate of chronic HCV infection. For examples, Tokushima (near Osaka, western Japan) is an area of high incidence of HCC and high prevalence of HCV infection in Japan. In Tokusima, 80% HCC cases were seropositive for anti-HCV, and 14% were seropositive for HBsAg [87]. In Osaka in western Japan, 90% of primary liver cancer cases are HCC, and 9% are cholangiocarcinoma [82]. The sex ratio of age-adjusted incidence rates (11.9 in females and 44.5 in males) of liver cancer in Osaka was 3.7 in the year 2002.

At any rate, most male-to-female ratios of the worldwide liver cancer incidence rates range from 2 to 4 not only in the high-risk areas, but in the low-risk areas as well.

7. LIVER CANCER INCIDENCE IN DIFFERENT ETHNIC GROUPS AND IMMIGRANT POPULATIONS

The incidence of liver cancer in populations by racial or ethnic origin in the United States is shown in Fig. **4** [82]. The lowest age-adjusted incidence rates are consistently found among Caucasian Americans (1.4 in females and 3.8 in males). Gradually increasing rates are found among the African American (2.1 in females and 7.1 in males), Japanese (4.3 in females and 5.5 in males), Filipino (2.4 in females and 10.9 in males), Hispanic Caucasian (3.8 in females and 10.6 in males), Chinese (5.0 in females and 16.2 in males), and Korean American (10.4 in females and 20.7 in males) populations. These cross-sectional rates are consistent with differences in risk factors and biological susceptibility to liver cancer across ethnic groups. Among females, the high-risk ethnic groups have a 2- to 5-fold higher incidence rate of liver cancer than that of the lowest-risk group Caucasian Americans. The male-to-female ratios in all the ethnic groups except for the Japanese-American populations are over 2 up to 4.5 (Fig. **4**). However, the incidence rates among Asians in the United States are evidently lower than those among native-born Asians in their homeland. In the United States, where approximately 85% of liver cancer cases are HCC, another study based on HCC incidence for the period 1973 to 1986 confirmed this notice. Age-adjusted HCC incidence rates among Chinese, Japanese, and Filipino immigrants to the United States and their descendants were generally lower than those among Asian residents born in Asia, and the sex ratios were constantly high [88].

These data show that the high sex ratios of HCC incidence rates among racial or ethnic groups and immigrant populations, whether born in high-risk areas or low-risk areas, are extremely consistent. Thus, the sex disparity in HCC incidence cannot completely be explained by the difference in exposures to environmental and lifestyle risk factors for HCC. Some mechanisms related to sex-associated difference of HCC incidence may be based on host-related biological factors including hormonal factors.

8. INCREASE OF HCC INCIDENCE RATES AMONG FEMALES AGED OVER 50 YEARS

Male sex, older age and cirrhosis are important host-related risk factors for the development of HCC (Table **5**). As mentioned above, the large majority of liver cancer cases occur in individuals with chronic HBV or

HCV infection. The mean age at onset of HBV-related HCC is around 55 years, which is 10 years younger than the average age at onset of HCV-related HCC [89]. Among patients with chronic hepatitis C or HCV-related cirrhosis, male sex and older age at diagnosis (>55 years) increase a 2- to 3-fold and a 2- to 4-fold risks of developing HCC, respectively [90-92]. Among patients with chronic hepatitis B or HBV-related cirrhosis, male sex and older age at diagnosis (>50 years) are also independent factors affecting progression to HCC [92,93].

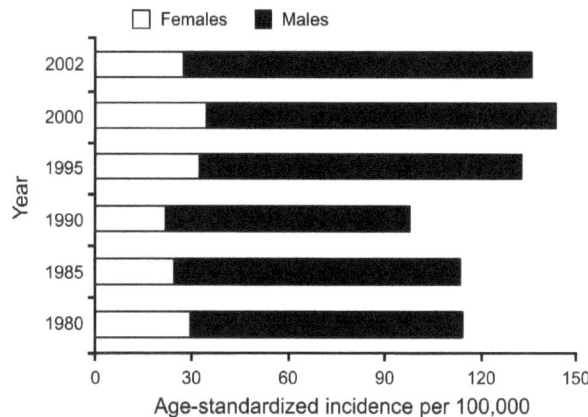

Fig. 4. Sex ratios of age-adjusted incidence rates of liver cancer by racial or ethnic group in the United States for the period 1993 to 1997 [82]. SEER, participants in the Surveillance, Epidemiology, and End Results (SEER) Program of the National Cancer Institute which covers over 14% of the United States population.

Table 5. Host-related major risk factors for development of HCC in cases with chronic HBV or HCV infection

Male sex	Up to 3-fold increased risk
Older age at diagnosis (>50 or 55 years)	Up to 4-fold increased risk
Cirrhosis	Up to 4-fold increased risk; 80%-90% of HCC cases in most populations

In the United States, HCC is rare among individuals younger than 40 years of age, and the greatest increase of HCC incidence occurs in cases 45 to 55 years of age [76]. The age-specific HCC incidence rates among females and males of African Americans and Caucasian Americans in the United States in the most recent time period, 1996 to 2000 [94], show that African Americans had an age-adjusted HCC incidence rate twice that of Caucasian Americans. The sex ratios of the HCC incidence rate were 3.4 for African Americans and 3.8 for Caucasian Americans in the period 1996 to 2000. The HCC incidence curves of males of both ethnic groups represented a linear increase on the logarithmic scale with increasing age. Among Caucasian-American males, the curves plateaued at age ≥70 years. Among African-American males, the curves leveled off much earlier, at age ≥55 years. In contrast to the linear increase of the incidence curves at the younger ages among males, the curves among females of both ethnic groups increased rapidly after ages 55 to 59 years, reaching peak levels at ages 80 to 84 years. These data indicate that HCC incidence rates among American females increase rapidly after age of 55 years.

In high-risk countries, sex ratios of HCC incidence tend to be higher, and the male excess is more pronounced below 50 years of age. Immigrant populations also show a shift in the sex ratio values. Japanese populations in the United States show a fairly stable sex ratio between 2 and 3 in the age groups above 50 years. Among Japanese-American females below age 50 years, however, the HCC incidence is too rare, and the sex ratio calculations are unreliable [75]. In Japan, Japanese populations show the male-to-female ratios of age-adjusted HCC incidence rates ranging from 6 to 7 in the age groups 40 to 55 years, whereas, in the age groups above 55 years, the incidence rates among females markedly increase with the less male excess and the sex ratios range between 2 and 5 [82]. These data suggest that Japanese females aged below 50 or 55 years are less vulnerable to HCC.

In Tokushima, Japan, a study on the age-specific sex ratios among Japanese HCC patients with HCV-related cirrhosis (n=1199) and chronic HBV infection (n=901) also confirmed the marked increase of HCC incidence rates among females aged 50 years and older. When the HCC patients were divided at diagnosis into two age groups, based on whether they are younger or older than the average menopausal age of 50 years, the older groups (≥50 years) with HCV (30.0%) and HBV (32.8%) infections had a 2- to 3-fold higher proportion of females than the younger groups (<50 years) with HCV (15.0%) and HBV (10.5%) infections [95,96] (Fig. **5**). These data show that cases of female sex and under 50 years old, namely "premenopausal women" are least vulnerable to HCC.

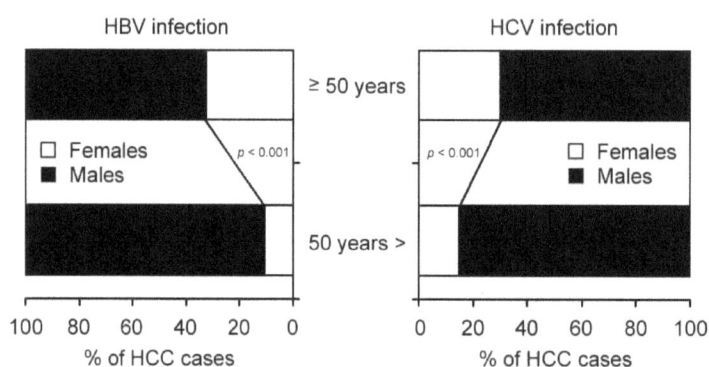

Fig. 5. Comparison of sex ratios between younger (<50 years) and older (≥50 years) groups of HBV-related HCC patients (left panel) and HCV-related HCC patients (right panel). Japanese individuals with HBV-related HCC were seropositive for HBsAg and seronegative for anti-HCV, and HCV-related individuals were seropositive for anti-HCV and seronegative for HBsAg, and. HCC was detected for the period 1994 to 2006 for HBV-related individuals [96], and 1993 to 2000 for HCV-related individuals [95] in Tokushima, Japan.

In Taiwan, where HBV infectin is hyper-endemic, a study of female persons on associations between natural or artificial menopause and HCC showed that the HCC risk was inversely related to the age at natural menopause. Ovariectomy performed at age 50 years or younger during premenopausal years was also a risk factor for HCC [97]. These data show that HCC incidence of female persons increase after menopause, suggesting that biological factors including estrogen-related sex hormone may play some role in the development of HCC and sex difference in HCC risk [98].

9. MAJORITY OF HCC CASES HAVE UNDERLYING CIRRHOSIS

The incidence of HCC is increasing in several developed countries. The trend is a result of a cohort effect related to infections with HBV and HCV, the incidence of which peaked in the 1950s to 1980s. Persistent these viral infections lead to chronic hepatitis and the end status of chronic hepatitis, cirrhosis. Cirrhosis from any cause predisposes to HCC and, thus, is considered a premalignant condition. Indeed, the majority of HCC patients worldwide have underlying cirrhosis. With the exception of some areas of the world where HBV infection is endemic and the role of other carcinogenic agents such as aflatoxin may be important, it is uncommon to find HCC in the absence of cirrhosis. HBV- or HCV-related chronic hepatitis and cirrhosis account for over 80% of HCC cases worldwide. In particular, cirrhosis of the end-stage of chronic hepatitis B or C represents the major known risk factors for HCC. Just like HCC as already noted, cirrhosis is largely a disease of men and postmenopausal women.

Table 6. Prevalence of major risk factors for HCC among cases with and without underlying cirrhosis [92]

% Among HCC Cases with Cirrhosis (80-90% of Total Cases)	Etiology	% Among HCC Cases without Cirrhosis (10-20% of Total Cases)
27-73	HCV infection	3-54
12-55	HBV infection	4-29
4-38	Heavy alcohol intake	0-28

The incidence of cirrhosis in cases with HCC is about 80%-90% in most populations, and, thus, approximately 10% to 20% of cases of HCC develop in individuals with chronic liver disease in the absence of cirrhosis (Table **6**). Among HCC cases with cirrhosis, HCV infection was identified in 27%-73%, HBV infection in 12%-55%, heavy alcohol intake in 4%-38%, and hemochromatosis (iron overload-related liver disease) and other causes in 2%-6%, leaving 4%-6% of the total number of cases without an identified cause. Among individuals with HCC but without underlying cirrhosis, HCV infection accounted for 3%-54%, HBV infection for 4%-29%, heavy alcohol intake for 0%-28%, and less common conditions for 1%-5% of the cases; in a variable proportion of HCC cases, the etiology was unknown. Overall, these studies show that HCC almost always occurs in a histologically abnormal liver and that the mere existence of chronic liver disease represents a potential risk for the development of HCC. Besides specific virus mechanisms that may contribute to carcinogenesis in the liver, chronic necroinflammation and generation of reactive oxygen species can induce chromosomal mutations and eventually malignant transformation of proliferating hepatocytes [92].

In Japanese studies, the summary HCC incidence rate was 1.8 per 100 person-years in cases with chronic hepatitis C in the absence of underlying cirrhosis at diagnosis and 7.1 in cases with cirrhosis. This shows a 4-fold higher risk of HCC for cases with cirrhosis than for those with chronic hepatitis C [92]. In the United States and Europe, the summary HCC incidence rate in cases with HCV-related cirrhosis was 3.7 per 100 person-years [92].

As with chronic HCV infection, the risk of HBV-related cirrhotic persons developing HCC is higher than that of persons with chronic hepatitis B without cirrhosis and appears to vary depending on geographic area. South-Eastern Asia, China, and sub-Saharan Africa, where HBV is hyper-endemic, have a high risk of HCC. In studies from Taiwan and Singapore, the summary HCC incidence rate was found to be 1.0 per 100 person-years in persons with chronic hepatitis B but without cirrhosis, and 3.2 in persons with HBsAg-related cirrhosis. In contrast, in studies from Europe, where HBV is low- or intermediate-endemic, the summary HCC incidence rate was 0.10 per 100 person-years in persons with chronic hepatitis B, and 2.2 in persons with cirrhosis. Thus, in areas of high HBV endemicity, individuals with cirrhosis have an approximately 3-fold higher risk for HCC than those with chronic hepatitis without cirrhosis; the corresponding figure in the West countries is approximately a 20-fold higher HCC risk [92].

Table 7. Male predominance of HCC risk in cirrhosis [99]

Study (Author, Year)	Country	Study Patients	Male-to-Female Ratio[a] (95% Confidence Interval)
Retrospective study (Ikeda, 2006 [100])	Japan	183 patients with HCV-related cirrhosis	1.6 (1.1-2.4)
Prospective study (Degos, 2000 [101])	France	416 patients with HCV-related cirrhosis	2.1 (1.2-3.9)
Prospective study (Chiaramonte, 1999 [102])	Italy	259 patients with HBV- and HCV-related cirrhosis	2.8 (1.5-5.3)
Prospective study (Bruno, 1997 [103])	Italy	163 patients with HCV-related cirrhosis	3.4 (1.3-9.3)
Retrospective study (Chiba, 1996 [104])	Japan	204 patients with HCV-related cirrhosis	4.2 (1.8-9.8)

[a]After adjustment for variables including age and/or markers of HBV or HCV infection.

In a retrospective study on the risk of HCC among persons with HCV-related cirrhosis in Japan, males still had a higher risk for HCC than females (odds ratio, an estimate of relative risk, 4.2; 95% confidence interval, 1.8-9.8) after adjustment for age, antibodies against HBV, and habitual alcohol drinking [104] (Table **7**). Similar findings have been reported in a prospective study with a mean follow-up of 5.7 years on HCC risk among 163 persons with HCV-related cirrhosis, showing a male-to-male ratio (95% confidence interval) of 3.4 (1.3-9.3) in Italy [103]. A retrospective study looks backwards and examines exposures to suspected risk or protection factors in relation to an outcome that is established at the start of the study. In contrast, a prospective study watches for outcomes, such as the development of a disease, during the study period and relates this to other factors such as suspected risk or protection factor(s). Prospective studies usually have fewer potential sources of bias and confounding than retrospective studies. In retrospective studies the odds ratio provides an estimate of relative risk. In another prospective study on 259 cirrhotic persons with a mean follow-up of 5.4 years in Italy, the HCC risk is higher in males than females (male-to-male ratio, 2.8; 95% confidence interval, 1.5-5.3) after adjustment for age and serostatus of HBsAg and anti-HCV [102]. Several other studies also show male predominance of HCC among cirrhotic persons consistently [100,101].

10. CONCLUSION

Male sex, older age and cirrhosis are important host-related risk factors for the development of HCC. In general, males have a greater risk of exposure to hepatitis viruses as well as a greater opportunity for drinking. Environmental factors may result in a higher preponderance of nutritional and exercise-associated problems in males. Being female or male is an important basic human variable that affects health and liver disease throughout the life span. Sex is defined as female or male according to their biological functions, while gender is shaped by environment and experience. A better understanding the physiopathogenesis of the sex-associated differences in chronic liver disease such as cirrhosis and HCC is important to developing new approaches to prevention, diagnosis, and treatment.

REFERENCES

[1]   Takano S, Yokosuka O, Imazeki F, *et al.* Incidence of hepatocellular carcinoma in chronic hepatitis B and C: a prospective study of 251 patients. Hepatology 1995;21:650-5.

[2]   Shiratori Y, Shiina S, Imamura M, *et al.* Characteristic difference of hepatocellular carcinoma between hepatitis B- and C- viral infection in Japan. Hepatology 1995;22:1027-33.

[3]   Zaman SN, Melia WM, Johnson RD, *et al.* Risk factors in development of hepatocellular carcinoma in cirrhosis: prospective study of 613 patients. Lancet 1985;1:1357-60.

[4]   Villa E, Baldini GM, Pasquinelli C, *et al.* Risk factors for hepatocellular carcinoma in Italy. Male sex, hepatitis B virus, non-A non-B infection, and alcohol. Cancer 1988;62:611-5.

[5]   Shimizu I, Inoue H, Yano M, *et al.* Estrogen receptor levels and lipid peroxidation in hepatocellular carcinoma with hepatitis C virus infection. Liver 2001;21:342-9.

[6]   Yeo AE, Matsumoto A, Shih JW, *et al.* Prevalence of hepatitis G virus in patients with hemophilia and their steady female sexual partners. Sex Transm Dis 2000;27:178-82.

[7]   Nolen-Hoeksema S. Gender differences in risk factors and consequences for alcohol use and problems. Clin Psychol Rev 2004;24:981-1010.

[8]   Tohme RA, Holmberg SD. Is sexual contact a major mode of hepatitis C virus transmission? Hepatology 2010;52:1497-505.

[9]   Shimizu I. Menopause-associated difference in chronic liver disease. In: Michalski J, Nowak I, eds. Menopause: Vasomotor Symptoms, Systematic Treatments ans Self-Care Measures, Hauppauge, New York: Nova Science, 2010:1-54.

[10]   Elbers JM, Asscheman H, Seidell JC, Gooren LJ. Effects of sex steroid hormones on regional fat depots as assessed by magnetic resonance imaging in transsexuals. Am J Physiol 1999;276:E317-E325.

[11]   Clark JM, Diehl AM. Defining nonalcoholic fatty liver disease: implications for epidemiologic studies. Gastroenterology 2003;124:248-50.

[12]   Shimizu I. Menopause-associated difference in chronic liver disease. In: Michalski J, Nowak I, eds. Menopause: Vasomotor Symptoms, Systematic Treatments ans Self-Care Measures, Hauppauge, New York: Nova Science, 2010:1-54.

[13]   WHO. Hepatitis B fact sheet. http://www.who.int/mediacentre/factsheets/fs204/en/. 2008.

[14]   WHO. Hepatitis C: global prevalence. Wkly Epidemiol Rec 1997;72:341-4.

[15]   National Center for Preparedness DaCoID. CDC Health Information for International Trabel 2008. Amsterdam: Elsevier Publishing, 2008.

[16] Lee WM. Hepatitis B virus infection. N Engl J Med 1997;337:1733-45.

[17] Alter MJ. Epidemiology of viral hepatitis and HIV co-infection. J Hepatol 2006;44:S6-S9.

[18] Yeo AE, Matsumoto A, Shih JW, *et al.* Prevalence of hepatitis G virus in patients with hemophilia and their steady female sexual partners. Sex Transm Dis 2000;27:178-82.

[19] Seeff LB, Beebe GW, Hoofnagle JH, *et al.* A serologic follow-up of the 1942 epidemic of post-vaccination hepatitis in the United States Army. N Engl J Med 1987;316:965-70.

[20] Lok AS, McMahon BJ. Chronic hepatitis B. Hepatology 2001;34:1225-41.

[21] Lok AS. Chronic hepatitis B. N Engl J Med 2002;346:1682-3.

[22] Donato F, Boffetta P, Puoti M. A meta-analysis of epidemiological studies on the combined effect of hepatitis B and C virus infections in causing hepatocellular carcinoma. Int J Cancer 1998;75:347-54.

[23] Seeff LB. Natural history of chronic hepatitis C. Hepatology 2002;36:S35-S46.

[24] El-Serag HB. Hepatocellular carcinoma and hepatitis C in the United States. Hepatology 2002;36:S74-S83.

[25] Kiyosawa K, Umemura T, Ichijo T, *et al.* Hepatocellular carcinoma: recent trends in Japan. Gastroenterology 2004;127:S17-S26.

[26] Davis GL, Dempster J, Meler JD, *et al.* Hepatocellular carcinoma: management of an increasingly common problem. Proc (Bayl Univ Med Cent) 2008;21:266-80.

[27] Brunetto MR, Oliveri F, Coco B, *et al.* Outcome of anti-HBe positive chronic hepatitis B in alpha-interferon treated and untreated patients: a long term cohort study. J Hepatol 2002;36:263-70.

[28] Hsu YS, Chien RN, Yeh CT, *et al.* Long-term outcome after spontaneous HBeAg seroconversion in patients with chronic hepatitis B. Hepatology 2002;35:1522-7.

[29] Bortolotti F, Jara P, Crivellaro C, *et al.* Outcome of chronic hepatitis B in Caucasian children during a 20-year observation period. J Hepatol 1998;29:184-90.

[30] Chan HL, Hui AY, Wong ML, *et al.* Genotype C hepatitis B virus infection is associated with an increased risk of hepatocellular carcinoma. Gut 2004;53:1494-8.

[31] Iloeje UH, Yang HI, Su J, *et al.* Predicting cirrhosis risk based on the level of circulating hepatitis B viral load. Gastroenterology 2006;130:678-86.

[32] Yang HI, Lu SN, Liaw YF, *et al.* Hepatitis B e antigen and the risk of hepatocellular carcinoma. N Engl J Med 2002;347:168-74.

[33] Sasaki T, Hattori T, Mayumi M. A large-scale survey on the prevalence of HBeAG and anti-HBe among asymptomatic carriers of HBV. Correlation with sex, age, HBsAG titre and s-GPT value. Vox Sang 1979;37:216-21.

[34] Zacharakis GH, Koskinas J, Kotsiou S, *et al.* Natural history of chronic HBV infection: a cohort study with up to 12 years follow-up in North Greece (part of the Interreg I-II/EC-project). J Med Virol 2005;77:173-9.

[35] Chisari FV, Ferrari C. Hepatitis B virus immunopathogenesis. Annu Rev Immunol 1995;13:29-60.

[36] Grossman CJ. Interactions between the gonadal steroids and the immune system. Science 1985;227:257-61.

[37] Blumberg BS, Sutnick AI, London WT, Melartin L. Sex distribution of Australia antigen. Arch Intern Med 1972;130:227-31.

[38] Furusyo N, Hayashi J, Sawayama Y, *et al.* Hepatitis B surface antigen disappearance and hepatitis B surface antigen subtype: a prospective, long-term, follow-up study of Japanese residents of Okinawa, Japan with chronic hepatitis B virus infection. Am J Trop Med Hyg 1999;60:616-22.

[39] Clerici E, Bergamasco E, Ferrario E, Villa ML. Influence of sex steroids on the antigen-specific primary antibody response *in vitro*. J Clin Lab Immunol 1991;34:71-8.

[40] Fung SK, Lok AS. Hepatitis B virus genotypes: do they play a role in the outcome of HBV infection? Hepatology 2004;40:790-2.

[41] Funk ML, Rosenberg DM, Lok AS. World-wide epidemiology of HBeAg-negative chronic hepatitis B and associated precore and core promoter variants. J Viral Hepat 2002;9:52-61.

[42] Hadziyannis SJ, Papatheodoridis GV. Hepatitis B e antigen-negative chronic hepatitis B: natural history and treatment. Semin Liver Dis 2006;26:130-41.

[43] Sjogren MH. Prevention of hepatitis B in nonresponders to initial hepatitis B virus vaccination. Am J Med 2005;118 Suppl 10A:34S-9S.

[44] McMahon BJ, Bruden DL, Petersen KM, *et al.* Antibody levels and protection after hepatitis B vaccination: results of a 15-year follow-up. Ann Intern Med 2005;142:333-41.

[45] Su FH, Chen JD, Cheng SH, *et al.* Seroprevalence of Hepatitis-B infection amongst Taiwanese university students 18 years following the commencement of a national Hepatitis-B vaccination program. J Med Virol 2007;79:138-43.

[46] McMahon BJ, Alberts SR, Wainwright RB, *et al.* Hepatitis B-related sequelae: prospective study in 1400 hepatitis B surface antigen-positive Alaska native carriers. Arch Intern Med 1990;150:1051-4.

[47] Fattovich G, Brollo L, Giustina G, *et al.* Natural history and prognostic factors for chronic hepatitis type B. Gut 1991;32:294-8.

[48] Zarski JP, Marcellin P, Leroy V, *et al.* Characteristics of patients with chronic hepatitis B in France: predominant frequency of HBe antigen negative cases. J Hepatol 2006;45:355-60.

[49] McMahon BJ. The natural history of chronic hepatitis B virus infection. Semin Liver Dis 2004;24 Suppl 1:17-21.

[50] Tanaka J, Kumagai J, Katayama K, *et al.* Sex- and age-specific carriers of hepatitis B and C viruses in Japan estimated by the prevalence in the 3,485,648 first-time blood donors during 1995-2000. Intervirology 2004;47:32-40.

[51] Murphy EL, Bryzman S, Williams AE, *et al.* Demographic determinants of hepatitis C virus seroprevalence among blood donors. JAMA 1996;275:995-1000.

[52] Yazdanpanah Y, De CG, Migueres B, *et al.* Risk factors for hepatitis C virus transmission to health care workers after occupational exposure: a European case-control study. Clin Infect Dis 2005;41:1423-30.

[53] Bakr I, Rekacewicz C, El HM, *et al.* Higher clearance of hepatitis C virus infection in females compared with males. Gut 2006;55:1183-7.

[54] Puoti C, Castellacci R, Montagnese F, *et al.* Histological and virological features and follow-up of hepatitis C virus carriers with normal aminotransferase levels: the Italian prospective study of the asymptomatic C carriers (ISACC). J Hepatol 2002;37:117-23.

[55] Jamal MM, Soni A, Quinn PG, *et al.* Clinical features of hepatitis C-infected patients with persistently normal alanine transaminase levels in the Southwestern United States. Hepatology 1999;30:1307-11.

[56] Boccato S, Pistis R, Noventa F, *et al.* Fibrosis progression in initially mild chronic hepatitis C. J Viral Hepat 2006;13:297-302.

[57] Tong MJ, el-Farra NS, Reikes AR, Co RL. Clinical outcomes after transfusion-associated hepatitis C. N Engl J Med 1995;332:1463-6.

[58] Poynard T, Ratziu V, Charlotte F, *et al.* Rates and risk factors of liver fibrosis progression in patients with chronic hepatitis C. J Hepatol 2001;34:730-9.

[59] Poynard T, Mathurin P, Lai CL, *et al.* A comparison of fibrosis progression in chronic liver diseases. J Hepatol 2003;38:257-65.

[60] Wright M, Goldin R, Fabre A, *et al.* Measurement and determinants of the natural history of liver fibrosis in hepatitis C virus infection: a cross sectional and longitudinal study. Gut 2003;52:574-9.

[61] Rodriguez-Torres M, Rios-Bedoya CF, Rodriguez-Orengo J, *et al.* Progression to cirrhosis in Latinos with chronic hepatitis C: differences in Puerto Ricans with and without human immunodeficiency virus coinfection and along gender. J Clin Gastroenterol 2006;40:358-66.

[62] uffic-Burban S, Poynard T, Valleron AJ. Quantification of fibrosis progression in patients with chronic hepatitis C using a Markov model. J Viral Hepat 2002;9:114-22.

[63] Gholson CF, Morgan K, Catinis G, *et al.* Chronic hepatitis C with normal aminotransferase levels: a clinical histologic study. Am J Gastroenterol 1997;92:1788-92.

[64] Renou C, Halfon P, Pol S, *et al.* Histological features and HLA class II alleles in hepatitis C virus chronically infected patients with persistently normal alanine aminotransferase levels. Gut 2002;51:585-90.

[65] Okanoue T, Makiyama A, Nakayama M, *et al.* A follow-up study to determine the value of liver biopsy and need for antiviral therapy for hepatitis C virus carriers with persistently normal serum aminotransferase. J Hepatol 2005;43:599-605.

[66] Strader DB, Wright T, Thomas DL, Seeff LB. Diagnosis, management, and treatment of hepatitis C. Hepatology 2004;39:1147-71.

[67] Conjeevaram HS, Fried MW, Jeffers LJ, *et al.* Peginterferon and ribavirin treatment in African American and Caucasian American patients with hepatitis C genotype 1. Gastroenterology 2006;131:470-7.

[68] Nagoshi S. Sex- or gender-specific medicine in hepatology. Hepatol Res 2008;38:219-24.

[69] Poynard T, Marcellin P, Lee SS, *et al.* Randomised trial of interferon alpha2b plus ribavirin for 48 weeks or for 24 weeks versus interferon alpha2b plus placebo for 48 weeks for treatment of chronic infection with hepatitis C virus. International Hepatitis Interventional Therapy Group (IHIT). Lancet 1998;352:1426-32.

[70] Hayashi J, Kishihara Y, Ueno K, *et al.* Age-related response to interferon ?? treatment in women vs men with chronic hepatitis C virus infection. Arch Intern Med 1998;178:177-81.

[71] MacNaughton J, Banah M, McCloud P, *et al.* Age related changes in follicle stimulating hormone, luteinizing hormone, oestradiol and immunoreactive inhibin in women of reproductive age. Clin Endocrinol (Oxf) 1992;36:339-45.

[72] Ferlay J, Bray F, Pisani P, Parkin DM. GLOBOCAN 2002: Cancer incidence, mortality and prevalence worldwide, IARC Cancer Base No. 5 Version 2.0. Lyon, France: IARC Press, 2004.

[73] World Health Organization. Mortality Database, WHO Statistical Information System. Available at http://www who int/whosis/en/ 2008.

[74] Coleman MP, Gatta G, Verdecchia A, *et al.* EUROCARE-3 summary: cancer survival in Europe at the end of the 20th century. Ann Oncol 2003;14 Suppl 5:v128-v149.

[75] Bosch FX, Ribes J, Diaz M, Cleries R. Primary liver cancer: worldwide incidence and trends. Gastroenterology 2004;127:S5-S16.

[76] El-Serag HB, Davila JA, Petersen NJ, McGlynn KA. The continuing increase in the incidence of hepatocellular carcinoma in the United States: an update. Ann Intern Med 2003;139:817-23.

[77] Benhamiche AM, Faivre C, Minello A, *et al.* Time trends and age-period-cohort effects on the incidence of primary liver cancer in a well-defined French population: 1976-1995. J Hepatol 1998;29:802-6.

[78] McGlynn KA, Tsao L, Hsing AW, *et al.* International trends and patterns of primary liver cancer. Int J Cancer 2001;94:290-6.

[79] Taylor-Robinson SD, Foster GR, Arora S, *et al.* Increase in primary liver cancer in the UK, 1979-94. Lancet 1997;350:1142-3.

[80] Law MG, Roberts SK, Dore GJ, Kaldor JM. Primary hepatocellular carcinoma in Australia, 1978-1997: increasing incidence and mortality. Med J Aust 2000;173:403-5.

[81] Parkin DM, Ohshima H, Srivatanakul P, Vatanasapt V. Cholangiocarcinoma: epidemiology, mechanisms of carcinogenesis and prevention. Cancer Epidemiol Biomarkers Prev 1993;2:537-44.

[82] Cancer incidence in five continents. Vol. VIII. IARC Scientific Publications No. 155. Parkin, D. M., Whelan, S. L., Ferlay, J., Teppo, L., and Thomas, D. B. 2002. Lyon, France, IARC; International Association of Cancer Registries.

[83] Chen JG, Zhu J, Parkin DM, *et al.* Trends in the incidence of cancer in Qidong, China, 1978-2002. Int J Cancer 2006;119:1447-54.

[84] Kensler TW, Qian GS, Chen JG, Groopman JD. Translational strategies for cancer prevention in liver. Nat Rev Cancer 2003;3:321-9.

[85] Yao DF, Horie C, Horie T, *et al.* Virological features of hepatitis C virus infection in patients with liver diseases in the inshore area of the Yangtze River. Tokushima J Exp Med 1994;41:49-56.

[86] Shimizu I, Yao D-F, Horie C, *et al.* Mutations in a hydrophilic part of the core gene of hepatitis C virus in patients with hepatocellular carcinoma in China. J Gastroenterol 1997;32:47-55.

[87] Shimizu I, Ito S. Hepatitis and hepatocellular carcinoma. Shikoku Acta Medica 2005;61:147-54.

[88] Rosenblatt KA, Weiss NS, Schwartz SM. Liver cancer in Asian migrants to the United States and their descendants. Cancer Causes Control 1996;7:345-50.

[89] Lee HS, Han CJ, Kim CY. Predominant etiologic association of hepatitis C virus with hepatocellular carcinoma compared with hepatitis B virus in elderly patients in a hepatitis B-endemic area. Cancer 1993;72:2564-7.

[90] Velazquez RF, Rodriguez M, Navascues CA, *et al.* Prospective analysis of risk factors for hepatocellular carcinoma in patients with liver cirrhosis. Hepatology 2003;37:520-7.

[91] Iwasaki Y, Takaguchi K, Ikeda H, *et al.* Risk factors for hepatocellular carcinoma in Hepatitis C patients with sustained virologic response to interferon therapy. Liver Int 2004;24:603-10.

[92] Fattovich G, Stroffolini T, Zagni I, Donato F. Hepatocellular carcinoma in cirrhosis: incidence and risk factors. Gastroenterology 2004;127:S35-S50.

[93] Tanaka Y, Mukaide M, Orito E, *et al.* Specific mutations in enhancer II/core promoter of hepatitis B virus subgenotypes C1/C2 increase the risk of hepatocellular carcinoma. J Hepatol 2006;45:646-53.

[94] McGlynn KA, Tarone RE, El-Serag HB. A comparison of trends in the incidence of hepatocellular carcinoma and intrahepatic cholangiocarcinoma in the United States. Cancer Epidemiol Biomarkers Prev 2006;15:1198-203.

[95] Shimizu I, Inoue H, Yano M, *et al.* Estrogen receptor levels and lipid peroxidation in hepatocellular carcinoma with hepatitis C virus infection. Liver 2001;21:342-9.

[96] Shimizu I, Kohno N, Tamaki K, *et al.* Female hepatology: favorable role of estrogen in chronic liver disease with hepatitis B virus infection. World J Gastroenterol 2007;13:4295-305.

[97]   Yu MW, Chang HC, Chang SC, *et al.* Role of reproductive factors in hepatocellular carcinoma: Impact on hepatitis B- and C-related risk. Hepatology 2003;38:1393-400.

[98]   Shimizu I. Impact of estrogens on the progression of liver disease. Liver Int 2003;23:63-9.

[99]   Chen CF, Yang HI, Chang HC, Chien-Jen Chen CJ. Gender difference in hepatocellular carcinoma associated with chronic hepatitis B and C. In: Shimizu I, ed. Female Hepatology: Impact of female sex against progression of liver disease, Kerala, India: Research Signpost, 2009.

[100] Ikeda K, Arase Y, Saitoh S, *et al.* Prediction model of hepatocarcinogenesis for patients with hepatitis C virus-related cirrhosis. Validation with internal and external cohorts. J Hepatol 2006;44:1089-97.

[101] Degos F, Christidis C, Ganne-Carrie N, *et al.* Hepatitis C virus related cirrhosis: time to occurrence of hepatocellular carcinoma and death. Gut 2000;47:131-6.

[102] Chiaramonte M, Stroffolini T, Vian A, *et al.* Rate of incidence of hepatocellular carcinoma in patients with compensated viral cirrhosis. Cancer 1999;85:2132-7.

[103] Bruno S, Silini E, Crosignani A, *et al.* Hepatitis C virus genotypes and risk of hepatocellular carcinoma in cirrhosis: a prospective study. Hepatology 1997;25:754-8.

[104] Chiba T, Matsuzaki Y, Abei M, *et al.* Multivariate analysis of risk factors for hepatocellular carcinoma in patients with hepatitis C virus-related liver cirrhosis. J Gastroenterol 1996;31:552-8.

CHAPTER 2

Gender Difference in Clinicopathologic Features and Prognosis of Patients with Hepatocellular Carcinoma

Pisit Tangkijvanich[1], Kittiyod Poovorawan[2] and Yong Poovorawan[3*]

[1]Department of Biochemistry, [2]Department of Medicine, and [3]Center of Excellence in Clinical Virology, Faculty of Medicine, Chulalongkorn University, Bangkok 10330, Thailand

Abstract: Hepatocellular carcinoma (HCC) occurs more frequently in males than in females, particularly in high- and intermediate-prevalence areas of the world. Accumulating data have shown that male patients tend to display more aggressive tumor characteristics than female patients at initial presentation. Moreover, the rate of spontaneous survival and survival after treatment is significantly lower in male patients with HCC. The explanation underlying gender disparity in clinicopathologic features and prognosis of the patients remains to be elucidated. Gender-specific lifestyle and social environment, as well as the role of sex hormones in hepatic carcinogenesis, may contribute to the observed gender difference in clinicopathologic aspects of HCC. In this review, we have summarized the clinicopathologic characteristics and survival of patients with HCC in relation to gender.

Keywords: Female, male, gender, liver cancer, hepatocellular carcinoma, hepatitis B, hepatitis C, alcohol, sex hormone, clinical feature, pathology, biological difference, prognosis, survival, carcinogenesis

1. INTRODUCTION

Hepatocellular carcinoma (HCC) is one of the most common cancers, which ranks fifth in males and eighth in females, and accounts for approximately 6% of all cancers worldwide [1]. The incidence of HCC is particularly high in areas where chronic hepatitis B virus (HBV) infection is prevalent. These regions include sub-Saharan Africa, the Far East and Southeast Asia where the annual rate of HCC exceeds 10 cases per 100,000 persons. In parts of China the annual incidence rate of HCC surpasses 30 cases per 100,000 persons. In Thailand, HCC represents the most common malignancy in males and the third most common malignancy in females. It has been estimated that more than 10,000 new cases of HCC are diagnosed each year, with an annual incidence of 6.8 per 100,000 in males and 2.3 per 100,000 in females [2]. In contrast, in low-incidence areas such as some parts of Europe and North America, the annual rate is less than 5 cases per 100, 000 persons [1].

Hepatic carcinogenesis is a multistage process with a multi-factorial etiology, including genetic and environmental interactions. The two most common risk factors are chronic infections with HBV and hepatitis C virus (HCV), which account for more than 50% and 20% of all HCC cases worldwide, respectively [3]. At present, chronic HBV infection continues to be the major risk factor; however, its significance is expected to decrease in the coming decades due to the universal vaccination of newborns. Chronic HCV infection has been the main cause of HCC in North America, Europe and Japan [4]. A meta-analysis has shown that co-infection with HBV and HCV is associated with a higher risk of developing HCC, suggesting a synergistic effect of the two infections in hepatic carcinogenesis. In cases positive for HBsAg and anti-HCV, the odds ratio (OR) is 22.5 [95% confidence interval (CI) = 19.5–26.0] and 17.3 (95% CI = 13.9–21.6), respectively. In cases of co-infection the OR is dramatically increased to 165 (95% CI = 81.2–374) [5]. Besides hepatitis virus infection, a small proportion of HCC cases are caused by various chronic liver diseases, including alcohol, non-alcohol steatohepatitis (NASH), genetic hemochromatosis and other uncommon etiologies.

Generally, HCC develops from pre-existing cirrhosis in approximately 80-90%, with the annual risk of HCC occurrence in cirrhosis estimated at between 1-6% [1, 4]. Cirrhosis, however, is not the only

---

Address correspondence to Yong Poovorawan: Center of Excellence in Clinical Virology, Faculty of Medicine, Chulalongkorn University, Bangkok 10330, Thailand; Tel: +662-256-4909; Fax: +662-256-4929; E-mail: yong.p@chula.ac.th

predisposing factor for the development of HCC because approximately 10-20% patients with chronic HBV infection do not have pre-existing cirrhosis. In the presence of cirrhosis, increasing age and male gender are independent risk factors for HCC. For instance, it has been estimated that a male Asian chronically-infected with HBV has a 20-25% lifetime risk of developing HCC [6]. The higher incidence of HCC in older age groups is likely related to the longer duration of chronic liver disease. For example, in high-prevalence areas, such as Southeast Asia and Africa, rates of HCC increase with age and reach a plateau at around 50 years of age [7]. In addition, the age-specific incidence rates also reflect the differences in etiology of HCC. In Thailand, the average age at onset of HBV-related HCC is around 50 years, which is approximately 10 years younger than the mean age at onset of HCV-related liver cancer [8, 9]. In Korea, the mean ages of HBV- and HCV-related HCC are approximately 55 and 65 years, respectively [10].

In contrast, although a predominance of HCC incidence among males has been well documented, the explanation of increased risk and unfavorable prognosis of liver cancer among men is less clear. Such a disparity may be due to a variety of mechanisms, ranging from gender-specific lifestyle and behavioral causes such as alcohol abuse and smoking to carcinogenic effects of sex hormones. In this review, we have summarized the clinicopathologic characteristics and survival of patients with HCC in relation to gender.

2. GENDER-RELATED INCIDENCE OF HCC

Various types of cancer occur more frequently in male than in female patients. In fact, it has long been recognized that females are less susceptible to cancers at sites that are conventional target organs of sex hormones. Such disparity is also the case with HCC. In all areas of the world, marked male predominance in HCC incidence is observed in both high- and low-risk areas, regardless of ethnic and geographic diversity [11]. Overall, the ratios in the gender-specific incidence rates of HCC vary from 2:1 to 8:1 in most series. In high- and intermediate-prevalence countries, gender ratios tend to be higher, and the male predominance is more pronounced below 50 years of age. For example, the sex ratio (males: females) is approximately 6:1 and 4:1 in Thailand and Korea, respectively [4, 9]. Interestingly, the advantage for females is attenuated after menopause, with an increased incidence of cirrhosis and liver cancer in older females [12]. In fact, the risk of HCC in females seems to be inversely related to the age of menopause, whereas postmenopausal hormone therapy could be a protective factor of HCC development [13]. In contrast, HCC is more equally distributed among males and females in low-prevalence areas, where the highest gender ratios occur later, in the 60–70-year age group. Interestingly, immigrant populations to low-prevalence areas also demonstrate a shift in the sex ratio. For example, Japanese populations in the United States exhibit a stable gender ratio (males: females) of 2-3:1 in the age groups above 50 years, whereas Japanese populations in Japan have an increased ratio of 3-5:1 in the same age groups. In the age groups below 50 years, the gender ratio of HCC among Japanese populations in Japan is approximately 7-10:1, while the incidence among women below the age of 50 years in the United States is extremely rare [14].

Not only limited to the incidence, males are predominantly affected with HCC-related mortalities, particularly in high- and intermediate-prevalence areas. In fact, the rate of spontaneous survival and survival after treatment is lower in males with HCC. However, when the mortality is expressed as proportion of all cancer mortality for a given region, the sex ratio tends to be less pronounced, especially in intermediate- and low-prevalence countries. For example, in USA, sex ratio (males: females) incidence and mortality rate are decreasing from 2.8 to 1.3, respectively. These data indicate that, in general, males tend to have higher rates of various types of cancers than females [4].

3. MECHANISMS INVOLVED IN GENDER DISPARITY IN HCC

One explanation for the higher rate of HCC among males could be attributed to a predominance of certain etiologies in male hepatic carcinogenesis in that males are more likely to be infected with HBV and HCV. It has also been speculated that gender-specific lifestyle and social environment such as excessive alcohol consumption and more frequent smoking could contribute to the observed gender difference of HCC incidence. However, such lifestyle and environment do not seem to fully account for these gender differences. Current data have emerged that signals induced by sex hormones and the inflammatory response might be an essential element of hepatic carcinogenesis [15].

3.1. Role of Gender-Specific Lifestyle and Environmental Factors

Consistent with the higher incidence of HCC in males than in females, a gender disparity in progression of chronic liver disease has been hypothesized [16]. The effects of gender on clinical features are particularly recognized both for HBV- and HCV-related chronic hepatitis. Males with chronic HBV infection are at higher risk of developing HCC compared with females. Two Taiwanese studies that included more than 3650 and 3930 participants with chronic HBV infection for a mean of approximately 11 and 12 years, respectively found that the adjusted relative risk for developing HCC in males was 2.1 (95% CI=1.3–3.3) and 3.6 (95% CI=2.4–5.3) compared with females [17, 18]. In fact, the sex difference becomes apparent in patients with chronic hepatitis B starting from the stage of early chronic infection. For example, the male to female ratio increased from 1.2 in asymptomatic carriers to 6.3 in chronic hepatitis and 9.8 in HCC in a Taiwanese study [19]. Male sex was identified as a risk factor for the reactivation of HBV in patients with HBeAg-negative chronic hepatitis, which might result in a higher incidence for progression to cirrhosis and HCC [20]. In addition, the results from long-term cohort studies conducted in different endemic areas of HBV have demonstrated that a lower percentage of males achieve HBeAg and HBsAg seroconversion compared to females [21, 22], which supports the hypothesis that males might have a less active immune response against HBV infection than females. Additional evidence supporting this postulation stems from the observation that males who received HBV vaccination at birth and were followed for a long-term period had a higher rate of chronic HBV infection than females [23].

Several cross-sectional studies have investigated factors associated with progression of fibrosis in chronic HCV infection. Besides older age and excessive alcohol consumption, male gender has been consistently identified as a factor associated with an increased rate of fibrosis progression [24]. Despite a similar prevalence of HCV infection among genders, numerous reports have shown that males progress faster to cirrhosis and have an increased risk of HCC [24]. For example, Poynard *et al.* have previously reported that host factors such as age at infection above 40 years, daily alcohol consumption of at least 50 g and male gender are strongly associated with fibrosis progression. In this study, the risk of progression has remained 2.5-fold higher in males than in females after controlling for other factors such as alcohol consumption, obesity and iron overload [25]. In addition, a French study has suggested that this gender disparity in fibrosis progression may be due to a protective effect of estrogen because postmenopausal women had increased rates of fibrosis progression and the use of hormone replacement therapy could reduce this rate [26]. Male patients chronically-infected with HCV are also less responsive to IFN-based therapy and have a higher incidence of early decompensation [25].

Hence, it seems that the predisposition of males for hepatic carcinogenesis in patients with chronic hepatitis B or C starts early in the course of chronic viral infection. Recent studies in hepatoma cell lines have suggested that the interaction between viral proteins and sex hormone receptors may play a role in viral-induced hepatic carcinogenesis [27]. For example, an interaction between the androgen pathway and hepatitis B x (HBx) protein, a multifunctional protein that is involved in hepatic carcinogenesis, has been recently established. It has been shown that the HBx protein can enhance the transcriptional activity of the androgen receptor (AR) in a ligand concentration-dependent manner, mainly through its effects on the c-Src and glycogen synthase kinase (GSK)-3β signaling pathways [28]. As a result, the augmentation of the AR pathway is likely more profound in male patients with chronic hepatitis B, which may explain the gender disparity in HBV-related HCC.

In general, the prevalence of heavy alcohol consumption is significantly different, being higher in males than in females. Heavy alcohol consumption, defined as ingestion of >50–70 g/day for prolonged periods, has long been recognized as a risk factor for developing HCC. Although its role in direct hepatic carcinogenesis is uncertain, it has been speculated that alcohol could be involved in the development of HCC through both direct and indirect mechanisms. An indirect mechanism includes the development of cirrhosis, which is the final common pathway to hepatic carcinogenesis [29]. In addition, chronic alcohol abuse might accelerate cancer development in some cases with HBV- or HCV-associated cirrhosis. In a case-control study, it has been demonstrated that among alcohol drinkers, the risk of HCC increased with increasing levels of alcohol intake with daily intake >60 g. In addition, a synergism between alcohol intake and hepatitis virus infections has become evident, with a more than additive but less than multiplicative increase in risk [30]. Several epidemiologic studies have also shown that the prevalence of chronic HBV and HCV infections were relatively high in patients with HCC who were alcoholics, suggesting a complex interaction between alcohol consumption and chronic viral hepatitis in the etiology of HCC [31]. Thus, it is reasonable to speculate that chronic alcohol abuse might accelerate cancer development in some cases with HBV- or HCV-associated cirrhosis and this may be partially responsible for the male preponderance of HCC in most series.

3.2. Role of Sex Hormones

It has been reported that DNA synthesis was more pronounced in male than in female cirrhosis patients and this might be one of the possible explanations for the gender discrepancy in HCC [32]. However, in patients who had already developed HCC, a significant difference in tumor cell proliferation between male and female patients was not detected [33]. A possible role for sex hormones in the development of HCC has also been implicated, although the underlying molecular mechanisms remain largely unknown [27, 34, 35]. Interestingly, the gender difference of HCC occurrence has also been noted in a diethylnitrosamine (DEN)-induced mouse model, with tumors developing more frequently in male than in female mice [36]. DEN is converted by liver enzymes to an electrophilic form, which damages DNA of the hepatocytes and induces liver regeneration, which subsequently leads to the development of HCC. In animal models, castration or administration of estrogens could protect male mice from tumor development, while ovariectomy increased the susceptibility to HCC in female mice [37]. Studies from animal models have also implicated that the hormonal effect may be related to testosterone's ability to enhance transforming growth factor (TGF)-α related hepatic carcinogenesis and hepatocyte proliferation [38]. Based on experimental studies, it has been postulated that androgen and estrogen contribute to the gender difference of HCC, but with distinct roles in each gender [34]. In brief, the higher activity of the androgen pathway functions as a tumor-promoting factor in male hepatic carcinogenesis, while the higher activity of the estrogen pathway acts as a tumor-suppressing factor in females.

Recently, Naugler *et al.* have suggested that indirect paracrine mechanisms are responsible for inhibition of hepatic carcinogenesis by estrogen [39]. In their report, it has been shown in a model of DEN-induced HCC that the tumor appeared in 100% of male but only in 13% female mice. Administration of DEN caused greater increases in serum interleukin (IL)-6 levels in male compared with female mice, suggesting that estrogen-mediated inhibition of the small adapter protein myeloid differentiation factor 88 (MyD-88)–dependent IL-6 produced by Kupffer cells could reduce HCC development in female mice. Tumor necrosis factor (TNF)-α, another pro-inflammatory cytokine also modestly accumulated after DEN administration, but no gender differences were observed and the ablation of TNF-α or its type I receptor did not affect IL-6 synthesis. Administration of estrogen to DEN-treated male mice decreased serum IL-6 levels and degree of liver damage. In addition, DEN-treated IL-6 knock-out mice had less liver injury and males exhibited a reduced incidence of HCC with disappearance of gender disparity, thus confirming a link between gender-dependent inflammatory responses and HCC development.

These data in animal models are consistent with findings in humans according to which postmenopausal women usually have persistent increases in pro-inflammatory cytokines, such as IL-6 and TNF-α as a result of the decline in ovarian function [40]. Indeed, susceptibility to HCC development tends to increase in such age groups compared to premenopausal females. A recent retrospective study in Japan has shown that higher serum IL-6 levels were considered to be an independent risk factor for HCC development in female but not male patients chronically-infected with hepatitis C. Thus, the measurement of serum IL-6 concentration may be useful in predicting the development of HCC in the future. However, the lower risk of progression to HCC in female patients could not be fully explained by estrogen-mediated inhibition of IL-6 production because a rather weak negative correlation was found between serum IL-6 and estradiol levels [41].

4. GENDER DIFFERENCE IN CLINICOPATHOLOGIC FEATURES OF HCC

In 2004, we retrospectively analyzed the clinicopathologic features at the time of diagnosis of 299 Thai patients with HCC in relation to gender (39 females and 260 males) [42]. As shown in Table **1**, the mean age of female patients (56.4 years) was slightly higher, but not significantly different from that of male patients (52.6 years). There was a significantly lower proportion of heavy alcohol consumption among females than males (P=0.002). However, there were neither significant differences in positive rates of serum HBsAg and anti-HCV, nor in the frequency of associated liver cirrhosis between the two groups. Similarly, no significant differences between groups were observed regarding mean serum alpha-fetoprotein (AFP) levels and biochemical abnormalities, with the exception that female patients had significantly lower serum bilirubin levels than male patients (P=0.03).

Table 1. Demographic and clinical data of female and male patients with HCC at initial diagnosis [42]

Characteristics	Female (n=39)	Male (n=260)	*p*
Age (years)	56.4±15.2	52.6±13.2	NS
Underlying cirrhosis (+:-)	36:3	251:9	NS
Viral hepatitis marker			
HBsAg (+:-)	18:21	147:113	NS
Anti-HCV (+:-)	5:34	23:237	NS
Heavy alcohol consumption (+:-)	3:36	83:177	0.002
Mean AFP (IU/ml)	48435.4±105231.6	40221.9±89147.9	NS
Biochemical liver function tests			
Total bilirubin (mg/dl)	1.5±1.2	3.1±2.3	0.03
Alkaline phosphatase (IU/L)	451.6±277.3	529.3±375.0	NS
AST (IU/L)	128.4±133.2	154.3±135.2	NS
ALT (IU/L)	62.7±52.6	87.6±97.5	NS
Albumin (g/dl)	3.6± 0.7	3.4±0.7	NS
Prothrombin time (sec)	14.5 ± 2.8	15.1±9.3	NS

Quantitative variables were expressed as mean ± SD; (+:-) indicates positive : negative.
NS = not significant.

Table **2** demonstrates the clinicopathologic data of the patients at the time of diagnosis of HCC. Female patients tended to have less aggressive tumor characteristics than male patients. For instance, the mean tumor size in females (8.6 cm) was significantly smaller than that of male patients (11.6 cm) (P=0.02). In addition, the nodular type of HCC appeared to be more frequently found among female patients, whereas the massive and diffuse types were more common among males (P=0.01). Furthermore, the tumors in the female group tended to be of a less advanced stage according to Okuda's criteria (P=0.04) and less' frequently associated with portal or hepatic vein invasion (P=0.03). It has been demonstrated that the presence of venous invasion is associated with a higher intrahepatic recurrence rate after the resection of the tumor [43]. Although HCC is characterized by its propensity for vascular invasion, it is interesting that in our study female patients with HCC had a much lower prevalence of venous involvement than males. However, no significant differences between groups were observed as to the degree of tumor differentiation, the prevalence of extrahepatic metastasis or ruptured HCC.

Similarly, there was no statistically significant difference between groups in terms of the number of patients treated with specific therapeutic modalities. However, female patients were more likely than male patients to undergo surgical resection, which included segmental and lobar resection, or to be treated with transcatheter arterial chemoembolization (TACE) (P=0.02 and 0.01, respectively). In contrast, a significantly higher proportion of male patients were treated with systemic chemotherapy than females (P=0.02). Thus, our study suggested that female patients tended to have a less advanced stage of HCC at initial diagnosis and, as a result, a higher proportion of cases were likely to undergo curative and palliative treatment, such as surgical resection or TACE, respectively.

Table 2. Clinicopathologic data of female and male patients with HCC at initial diagnosis [42]

Characteristics	Female (n=39)	Male (n=260)	p
Mean tumor size (cm)	8.1±3.9	11.6±4.5	0.02
Tumor size			
≤ 5 cm: >5cm	9:30	30:230	0.04
Gross appearance of HCC			
Nodular:Multinodular:Massive:Diffuse	12:10:14:3	30:52:115:63	0.01
Tumor cell differentiation			
Well:Moderately:Poorly	3:5:4	11:66:32	NS
Okuda' s staging (I:II:III)	13:23:3	43:180:37	0.04
Portal or hepatic vein invasion (+:-)	6:33	84:176	0.03
Extrahepatic metastasis (+:-)	5:34	37:223	NS
Ruptured HCC (+: -)	1:38	29:231	NS
Therapy for HCC (+:-)	22:17	105:155	NS
Modality of therapy			
Surgical resection (+:-)	9:30	27:233	0.02
Chemoembolization (+:-)	13:26	43:217	0.01
Systemic chemotherapy (+:-)	0:39	31:229	0.02

Quantitative variables were expressed as mean ± SD; (+:-) indicates positive : negative.

Cong *et al.* conducted a study in mainland China to compare the clinicopathologic characteristics of 104 female HCC patients who underwent surgical resection with those of 900 male HCC cases. Their data have shown that the development of HCC in females appeared at a younger age than that of HCC in males (mean age of 46 and 49 years, respectively) and usually was associated with a lower frequency of cirrhosis (49% and 68%, respectively) [44]. Dohmen *et al.* [45] retrospectively investigated 704 consecutive Japanese patients with HCC (217 females and 487 males) to determine clinicopathologic differences between males and females. Of the variables examined, the significant factors related to gender disparity in their study were tumor size, the number of tumors and the presence of portal vein thrombosis. However, no significant difference was identified in terms of underlying cirrhosis, which contrasted the data shown by Cong *et al.* In addition, no significant difference with respect to treatment modalities, such as surgical resection, percutaneous ethanol injection (PEI), radiofrequency ablation (RFA), TACE and chemotherapy was found between both genders.

Similarly, yet to be addressed are the effects of other tumor pathologic features, such as tumor encapsulation during the disease-free period after surgical resection of the tumor, which has been shown to be an independent favorable prognostic marker in HCC. Ng *et al.* [33] conducted a study in Hong Kong to examine the gender-related pathological characteristics of patients with HCC (35 females and 243 males), who had undergone surgical resection of the tumor. Their data have demonstrated that females had a significantly higher prevalence of tumor encapsulation than males (80% and 45%, respectively). Furthermore, the tumors in females were frequently less invasive in terms of lower prevalence of tumor microsatellites, liver invasion and positive histological margin. Tumor microsatellite formation was found in 16.1% of the tumors in females, compared with 59.7% in males *(P < 0.0001)*. In addition, liver invasion was found in 37% of tumors in women and in 61% in men *(P =0.03)*. Moreover, only 6.1% of tumors in females had a positive histological margin, compared to 24.1% in males *(P =0.04)*.

Benvegnu *et al.* [46] conducted a study to compare incidence, risk factors and morphologic pattern of HCC development in HBV- and HCV-related cirrhosis in an Italian population. According to their report, 401 patients had been prospectively followed by periodic ultrasound examination for 14-189 months. During follow-up, 77 (19.2%) patients developed HCC, with 5 and 10 years cumulative incidence of 10 and 27.5%, respectively. The risk of HCC was significantly higher in HBV and HCV co-infected patients (P=0.014) compared to those of mono-infection with HBV or HCV. The pattern of HCC diagnosed by ultrasound was categorized into nodular and infiltrating types, which were found in approximately 82% and 18%, respectively. Nodular HCC was associated with older age (P=0.0001), longer duration (P=0.002) and more advanced stage (P=0.0001) of cirrhosis but not with the viral etiology. In contrast, development of infiltrating HCC was unrelated to age and disease duration and stage, but was associated with male sex (P=0.01), HBV mono-infection (P=0.06) and HBV and HCV co-infection (P=0.0001).

Recently, Farinati *et al.* [47] used the ITA.LI.CA (Italian Liver Cancer) database, which included 1834 patients consecutively diagnosed with HCC (482 females, 1352 males) to determine whether female patients had more favorable prognostic factors than males. Their results showed that female patients were characterized by older age (P=0.0001), higher prevalence of HCV infection (P=0.0001), diagnosis more frequently by surveillance (P=0.003), higher AFP levels (P=0.0055), portal vein thrombosis (P=0.04), and extrahepatic metastasis (P=0.0001). In addition, HCC in females was more frequently unifocal (P=0.0001), smaller (P=0.001), well differentiated (P=0.001), and of lower Cancer of the Liver Italian Program (CLIP) and tumor-nodes-metastases (TNM) stage (P=0.0001 and 0.0001, respectively). Despite these clinical features at presentation, the same proportion of females underwent curative treatments (liver transplantation, surgical resection and percutaneous ablation) as males.

Lam *et al.* [48] retrospectively analyzed a total of 3,171 Chinese patients with HCC from 1989 to 2003 (520 females and 2651 males) to determine the influence of gender on clinicopathologic features and patient's survival. In this report, the mean age of female patients was approximately 4 years above that of male patients (60.8 and 56.5 years, respectively). There was no difference in the history of diabetes mellitus and family history of HCC in first degree relatives. However, chronic HBV infection was found more frequently in males, whereas chronic HCV infection was more predominant in females. Moreover, male patients were more likely to be smokers and alcohol drinkers. In this study, there were 946 patients having undergone curative treatment, 1,388 palliative treatment, and 837 supportive treatment. Although gender is an independent variable for survival after curative treatment, there was no difference in Child-Pugh status, tumor characteristics such as number of tumor nodules, size of tumor, major vascular invasion, invasion of adjacent organs, and tumor rupture, and the use of different treatments between both genders. However, as for cases undergoing curative treatment, there were more females at earlier stages of the disease compared with male patients.

Taken together, most reports indicate that female patients with HCC have certain clinicopathologic features different from those in male patients. In particular, HCC in females tends to exhibit less aggressive tumor characteristics and better prognostic factors at initial presentation. For example, HCC in females has a lower prevalence of portal vein thrombosis, extrahepatic metastasis and earlier stages of the cancer. Such disparity may be partly related to real biological differences of the cancer between genders as pointed out in the animal models. In addition, it is possible that the difference in tumor surveillance practices of females relative to their male counterparts may contribute to the earlier stages of disease and favorable clinicopathologic characteristics in female patients with HCC.

5. GENDER DIFFERENCE IN SURVIVAL OF HCC

Apart from generally recognizing the lower incidence of HCC in females, most available data have repeatedly reported that female HCC has a better survival prognosis compared with male patients. For example, a large–scale prospective cohort study in China demonstrated the survival benefit in female patients [49]. In addition, a survival benefit was particularly observed in females undergoing surgical resection. For instance, according to the study by Nagasue *et al.*, significantly better survival rates were found in females 4 years after hepatic surgery [50]. Cong *et al.* also demonstrated that the survival rates after surgery were approximately 50% and 25% in females and males, respectively [44]. Likewise, Lee *et al.* [51], reported that female cirrhosis patients with HCC had 5-year disease survival rates after hepatic resection, which was higher than in males (approximately 65% and 30%, respectively) [52]. Conversely, such favorable prognosis in females was not consistently observed among patients with inoperable tumors [42, 53-55].

Among these studies, however, there have been few reports that have specifically compared the influence of gender on natural history and prognosis of patients with HCC. Moreover, in several analyses of independent variables of prognosis, gender could not be demonstrated as an independent factor for survival in patients with HCC, who had undergone surgical resection [43, 56-59] or in those with inoperable tumors [53, 60].

Ng *et al.* [33] showed that females had a lower incidence of tumor recurrence after surgical resection, with median disease free survival of 19.5 months compared with 4.5 months for males (P < 0.001). Females also had more favorable actuarial survival than males [36.5 and 12.4 months, respectively (P = 0.002)]. They concluded that females with HCC, who underwent surgical resection had better survival prognosis and lower tumor recurrence than males. The better prognosis in females with HCC appeared to be related to certain pathologic characteristics of the tumor (*i.e.*, frequent encapsulation and lower tumor invasiveness).

In our study [42], the median survival time of Thai patients with HCC, regardless of their gender, was approximately 5 months. The Kaplan-Meier survival curves demonstrated that the overall median survival for female and male patients were approximately 14 and 4 months, respectively (P=0.004, using log-rank test). For patients who were treated with any specific therapeutic modality, the median survival for the female and male group were approximately 17 and 7 months, respectively (P=0.025). In the untreated cases, the median survival of the female group was longer than that of the male group (approximately 9 and 3 months, respectively), however, this difference did not reach statistical significance (P=0.24). Thus, better survival in females was observed in those who had undergone curative surgery or palliative treatment. It is well recognized that hepatic resection is one of the most effective therapeutic modalities offering a hope of cure for patients with HCC. Moreover, non-surgical approaches such as TACE appear to be beneficial in prolonging survival for some patients with inoperable tumors [61, 62]. As for untreated cases, the influence of gender on prognosis appeared to be limited since significant difference in survival between groups was not observed, although there was a trend for females to survive longer.

Univariate analysis of the main variables was performed to determine significant risk factors associated with the overall survival. In addition to male sex, high serum AFP levels, Okuda's stage II and III HCC, massive or diffuse types of tumors, tumor mass size exceeding 5 cm in diameter, venous invasion and extrahepatic metastasis, and an unfavorable prognosis were observed in patients who did not receive any specific therapy for HCC. Stepwise Cox regression multivariate analysis revealed that high serum AFP levels, venous invasion, extrahepatic metastasis and absence of specific therapy were significantly and independently predictive for unfavorable prognosis (Table **3**). Nonetheless, gender was not selected in the final analysis as an independent predictor of survival.

From our data, it could be speculated that the prognosis of HCC was not directly influenced by the gender of the patients, because gender was not selected as an independent predictor of survival from the multivariate analysis. A better prognosis in females was probably attributed to a less advanced stage of HCC at initial diagnosis and, as a result, a higher proportion of cases were likely to undergo curative or palliative therapies. In this study, for example, approximately 25% and 35% of female patients were treated with hepatic resection or TACE, respectively, while only approximately 10% and 15% of males underwent such therapeutic modalities. In addition to therapeutic factors, some pathologic features indicative of tumor invasiveness, such as venous involvement, appear to be significant factors influencing the survival of HCC. It seemed, therefore, that this was probably one of the main factors contributing to different survival rates between the two genders in our study. Thus, better prognosis in females might be related to more favorable tumor characteristics and less advanced stages at initial diagnosis. As a result, female patients were more likely than male patients to undergo hepatic resection or to receive palliative treatment.

Likewise, Dohmen *et al.* [45] demonstrated that there was a significant difference in survival between male and female patients with a 1-, 3-, 5- and 7-year survival estimate of 67.7, 40.6, 23.8 and 8.7% versus 73.5, 50.3, 26.3 and 15.4%, respectively (P=0.0167). The significant factors related to gender difference were age, tumor characteristics and the type of follow-up, which were divided into three categories: closely followed-up group by monthly AFP measurements and ultrasound at least every 4 months; a non-closely followed-up group; and an incidental group discovered from related symptoms. The detection rates of HCC throughout these three groups were 19.3%, 46.2% and 34.5% in males and 28.1%, 46.5% and 25.4% in females, respectively, which reached a significant difference between both genders (P-value=0.0097). Of particular importance in this report was that when patients' survival was compared in relation to the same tumor characteristics, such as in early HCC with less than 3 cm as the largest diameter or solitary HCC without portal thrombosis, there was no significant difference in survival observed between genders. Thus, it was concluded that the better survival of females in comparison to male patients with HCC might be related to the type of follow-up, which might contribute to a higher detection rate of less aggressive tumor characteristics.

Table 3. Independent predictors influencing survival in HCC in multivariate analysis

(Selected studies specifically compared the influence of gender on survival of patients) [42, 47, 48]

Variables	Hazard ratio (95% CI)	*P* value
Tangkijvanich *et al.*		
AFP (>400 ng/ml)	1.67 (1.03-2.71)	0.037
Major vascular invasion	1.73 (1.04-2.89)	0.035
Extrahepatic metastasis	2.37 (1.30-4.37)	0.005
No therapy	2.87 (1.63-5.04)	0.0002
Lam *et al.*		
Gender	ND (0.59-0.98)	0.034
ICG retention value at 15 min	ND (1.01-1.03)	0.000
Number of tumor nodules	ND (1.04-1.11)	0.000
Size of tumor	ND (1.04-1.08)	0.000
Major vascular invasion	ND (1.26-2.58)	0.001
Invasion of the adjacent organs	ND (1.34-2.68)	0.000
Tumor rupture	ND (1.41-2.54)	0.000
Farinati *et al.*		
Gender	0.84 (0.72-0.99)	0.042
Age	1.01 (1.00-1.02)	<0.001
Constitutional symptoms	1.51 (1.29-1.76)	<0.001
Child-Puge class	1.20 (1.03-1.41)	0.017
Number of lesions	1.14 (1.05-1.24)	0.001
Portal thrombosis	1.46 (1.16-1.84)	0.001
CLIP score	1.69 (1.60-1.77)	<0.001

CI, confident interval; AFP, Alpha-fetoprotein; ICG, Indocyanine green test;

ND, no data; CLIP, Cancer of the Liver Italian Program.

Data from Farinati *et al.* [47], which included a relatively large number of female HCC patients with adequate and long term follow-up, also demonstrated that females had less aggressive tumor characteristics and had a significantly better survival than males (median survival were 29 and 24 months, respectively, P=0.0001). This difference was less noticeable in patients who had undergone a tumor surveillance program before the diagnosis of HCC (median survival were 36 and 33 months, respectively, P>0.05). In contrast, when comparing between females undergoing surveillance with males diagnosed incidentally, a clear-cut statistically significant difference in survival was observed (median survival were 36 and 17 months, respectively, P<0.0001). In the Cox multivariate analysis, gender was identified as an independent predictor of survival (Table **3**). In concordance with Dohmen *et al.* [45] and our report [42], it has been speculated that the difference in prognosis of HCC between both genders was simply attributable to females being more compliant with surveillance and, consequently, the tumor could be detected at an earlier stage and the patients were offered more therapeutic options. Thus, such a lead-time bias in the diagnosis of HCC may account for the gender difference in prognosis rather than real biological differences of the tumor.

Lam *et al.* [48]. demonstrated that, although gender is an independent variable for survival, there was no difference in tumor characteristics and stages, as well as the modalities of treatment between both genders at initial presentation. In their study, the overall median survival of both genders irrespective of treatment was 1.5 months longer in females than in males (median survival of 8.9 vs. 7.4 months, respectively, P=0.004). However, when survival was analyzed in relation to treatment modality, a surplus of median survival of 25.7 months was observed in females undergoing curative treatment (median survival of 73.6 vs. 47.9 months, respectively, P = 0.007), but no significant difference after palliative or supportive treatment. When survival was analyzed in relation to stages of HCC, female patients at earlier stages also had a better survival than male patients at the same stages. For example, a clear survival benefit in females was observed in early-stage diseases among patients chronically infected with HBV (median survival of 96.4 vs. 47.9 months in females and males, respectively, P = 0.044). With multivariate analysis, gender, indocyanine green test value at 15 minutes, number of tumor nodules, size of tumor, major vascular invasion, invasion of adjacent organs, and tumor rupture were the independent variables for survival (Table **3**). These data supported the concept that better survival in female patients with HCC might be related to gender by itself because a lead-time bias in the diagnosis of the cancer, if present, was rather small.

In this study, history of using oral contraceptives was also an independent factor with survival benefit in female patients. To support this interesting finding, analysis of survival was compared between females not using oral contraceptives and male patients undergoing curative treatment. There was no significant survival benefit between females not using oral contraceptives and the male patients (median survival of 64.9 vs. 45.8 months, respectively, P=0.361). Although type of oral contraceptives and duration of use were not analyzed, these observations as an independent factor for survival benefit further support the postulation of a protective effect of estrogen in HCC development.

Taken together, with respect to gender disparity in survival, most reports have shown that female patients with HCC have a better prognosis than male patients, particularly those who had undergone curative treatment. The explanations of survival benefit in females may be partly related to a lead-time bias in the diagnosis of HCC, as females tend to be more compliant to cancer surveillance. However, the influence of gender, particularly a possible role of sex hormones in the development of HCC, may also account for the difference.

6. CONCLUSION

HCC is a predominantly male cancer, particularly in high- and intermediate-prevalence areas of the world. In addition, male patients tended to display more aggressive tumor characteristics than female patients at initial time of diagnosis of HCC. Moreover, the rate of spontaneous survival and survival after treatment is significant lower in males with HCC. The reasons underlying gender disparity in cancer incidence, as well as clinicopathologic features and prognosis are not completely clear. It has been speculated that gender-specific lifestyle and social environment may contribute to the observed gender difference of HCC incidence. In addition, emerging data from experimental studies have also suggested that signals induced by sex hormones and the inflammatory response appear to be crucial in hepatic carcinogenesis, which might result in the difference among genders with respect to clinicopathologic presentations and survival of patients with HCC. Finally, a lead-time bias in the diagnosis and management of HCC may also account for the gender difference in clinicopathologic characteristics and prognosis. Further well-designed experimental and clinical studies to verify the role of gender in the development of HCC and its clinical aspects are certainly needed to address this intriguing issue.

ACKNOWLEDGEMENTS

We would like to express our gratitude to the Commission on Higher Education, Ministry of Education, the Center of Excellence in Clinical Virology, Chulalongkorn University, CU Centenary Academic Development Project, King Chulalongkorn Memorial Hospital, the National Research University Project of CHE and the Ratchadaphiseksomphot Endowment Fund (HR1162A, HR1155A) and the Thailand Research Fund for their generous support. Finally we would like to thank Ms. Petra Hirsch for reviewing the manuscript.

REFERENCES

[1]   Sherman M. Hepatocellular carcinoma: epidemiology, surveillance, and diagnosis. Semin Liver Dis 2010;30:3-16.

[2]   Srivatanakul P. Epidemiology of Liver Cancer in Thailand. Asian Pac J Cancer Prev 2001;2:117-121.

[3]   Parkin DM, Bray F, Ferlay J, Pisani P. Estimating the world cancer burden: Globocan 2000. Int J Cancer 2001;94:153-6.

[4]   Nordenstedt H, White DL, El-Serag HB. The changing pattern of epidemiology in hepatocellular carcinoma. Dig Liver Dis 2010;42 Suppl 3:S206-14.

[5]   Donato F, Boffetta P, Puoti M. A meta-analysis of epidemiological studies on the combined effect of hepatitis B and C virus infections in causing hepatocellular carcinoma. Int J Cancer 1998;75:347-54.

[6]   Yu MW, Chang HC, Liaw YF, *et al.* Familial risk of hepatocellular carcinoma among chronic hepatitis B carriers and their relatives. J Natl Cancer Inst 2000;92:1159-64.

[7]   Bosch FX, Ribes J, Cleries R, Diaz M. Epidemiology of hepatocellular carcinoma. Clin Liver Dis 2005;9:191-211, v.

[8]   Tangkijvanich P, Anukulkarnkusol N, Suwangool P, *et al.* Clinical characteristics and prognosis of hepatocellular carcinoma: analysis based on serum alpha-fetoprotein levels. J Clin Gastroenterol 2000;31:302-8.

[9]   Tangkijvanich P, Hirsch P, Theamboonlers A, *et al.* Association of hepatitis viruses with hepatocellular carcinoma in Thailand. J Gastroenterol 1999;34:227-33.

[10]   Lee HS, Han CJ, Kim CY. Predominant etiologic association of hepatitis C virus with hepatocellular carcinoma compared with hepatitis B virus in elderly patients in a hepatitis B-endemic area. Cancer 1993;72:2564-7.

[11]   El-Serag HB. Hepatocellular carcinoma: an epidemiologic view. J Clin Gastroenterol 2002;35:S72-8.

[12]   Shimizu I, Ito S. Protection of estrogens against the progression of chronic liver disease. Hepatol Res 2007;37:239-47.

[13]   Yu MW, Chang HC, Chang SC, *et al.* Role of reproductive factors in hepatocellular carcinoma: Impact on hepatitis B- and C-related risk. Hepatology 2003;38:1393-400.

[14]   Bosch FX, Ribes J, Diaz M, Cleries R. Primary liver cancer: worldwide incidence and trends. Gastroenterology 2004;127:S5-S16.

[15]   Wands J. Hepatocellular carcinoma and sex. N Engl J Med 2007;357:1974-6.

[16]   Giannitrapani L, Soresi M, La Spada E, *et al.* Sex hormones and risk of liver tumor. Ann N Y Acad Sci 2006;1089:228-36.

[17]   Chen CJ, Yang HI, Su J, *et al.* Risk of hepatocellular carcinoma across a biological gradient of serum hepatitis B virus DNA level. JAMA 2006;295:65-73.

[18]   Chen CL, Yang HI, Yang WS, *et al.* Metabolic factors and risk of hepatocellular carcinoma by chronic hepatitis B/C infection: a follow-up study in Taiwan. Gastroenterology 2008;135:111-21.

[19]   Chu CM, Liaw YF, Sheen IS, *et al.* Sex difference in chronic hepatitis B virus infection: an appraisal based on the status of hepatitis B e antigen and antibody. Hepatology 1983;3:947-50.

[20]   Chu CM, Liaw YF. Incidence and risk factors of progression to cirrhosis in inactive carriers of hepatitis B virus. Am J Gastroenterol 2009;104:1693-9.

[21]   Zacharakis GH, Koskinas J, Kotsiou S, *et al.* Natural history of chronic HBV infection: a cohort study with up to 12 years follow-up in North Greece (part of the Interreg I-II/EC-project). J Med Virol 2005;77:173-9.

[22]   Alward WL, McMahon BJ, Hall DB, *et al.* The long-term serological course of asymptomatic hepatitis B virus carriers and the development of primary hepatocellular carcinoma. J Infect Dis 1985;151:604-9.

[23]   Su FH, Chen JD, Cheng SH, *et al.* Seroprevalence of Hepatitis-B infection amongst Taiwanese university students 18 years following the commencement of a national Hepatitis-B vaccination program. J Med Virol 2007;79:138-43.

[24]   Feld JJ, Liang TJ. Hepatitis C - identifying patients with progressive liver injury. Hepatology 2006;43:S194-206.

[25]   Poynard T, Bedossa P, Opolon P. Natural history of liver fibrosis progression in patients with chronic hepatitis C. The OBSVIRC, METAVIR, CLINIVIR, and DOSVIRC groups. Lancet 1997;349:825-32.

[26]   Di Martino V, Lebray P, Myers RP, *et al.* Progression of liver fibrosis in women infected with hepatitis C: long-term benefit of estrogen exposure. Hepatology 2004;40:1426-33.

[27]   Kalra M, Mayes J, Assefa S, *et al.* Role of sex steroid receptors in pathobiology of hepatocellular carcinoma. World J Gastroenterol 2008;14:5945-61.

[28]   Yang WJ, Chang CJ, Yeh SH, *et al.* Hepatitis B virus X protein enhances the transcriptional activity of the androgen receptor through c-Src and glycogen synthase kinase-3beta kinase pathways. Hepatology 2009;49:1515-24.

[29]   McKillop IH, Schrum LW. Role of alcohol in liver carcinogenesis. Semin Liver Dis 2009;29:222-32.

[30]   Donato F, Tagger A, Gelatti U, *et al*. Alcohol and hepatocellular carcinoma: the effect of lifetime intake and hepatitis virus infections in men and women. Am J Epidemiol 2002;155:323-31.

[31]   Di Bisceglie AM, Carithers RL, Jr., Gores GJ. Hepatocellular carcinoma. Hepatology 1998;28:1161-5.

[32]   Tarao K, Ohkawa S, Shimizu A, *et al*. The male preponderance in incidence of hepatocellular carcinoma in cirrhotic patients may depend on the higher DNA synthetic activity of cirrhotic tissue in men. Cancer 1993;72:369-74.

[33]   Ng IO, Ng MM, Lai EC, Fan ST. Better survival in female patients with hepatocellular carcinoma. Possible causes from a pathologic approach. Cancer 1995;75:18-22.

[34]   Yeh SH, Chen PJ. Gender disparity of hepatocellular carcinoma: the roles of sex hormones. Oncology 2010;78 Suppl 1:172-9.

[35]   Ruggieri A, Barbati C, Malorni W. Cellular and molecular mechanisms involved in hepatocellular carcinoma gender disparity. Int J Cancer 2010;127:499-504.

[36]   Rogers AB, Fox JG. Inflammation and Cancer. I. Rodent models of infectious gastrointestinal and liver cancer. Am J Physiol Gastrointest Liver Physiol 2004;286:G361-6.

[37]   Nakatani T, Roy G, Fujimoto N, *et al*. Sex hormone dependency of diethylnitrosamine-induced liver tumors in mice and chemoprevention by leuprorelin. Jpn J Cancer Res 2001;92:249-56.

[38]   Matsumoto T, Takagi H, Mori M. Androgen dependency of hepatocarcinogenesis in TGFalpha transgenic mice. Liver 2000;20:228-33.

[39]   Naugler WE, Sakurai T, Kim S, *et al*. Elsharkawy AM, Karin M. Gender disparity in liver cancer due to sex differences in MyD88-dependent IL-6 production. Science 2007;317:121-4.

[40]   Pfeilschifter J, Koditz R, Pfohl M, Schatz H. Changes in proinflammatory cytokine activity after menopause. Endocr Rev 2002;23:90-119.

[41]   Nakagawa H, Maeda S, Yoshida H, *et al*. Serum IL-6 levels and the risk for hepatocarcinogenesis in chronic hepatitis C patients: an analysis based on gender differences. Int J Cancer 2009;125:2264-9.

[42]   Tangkijvanich P, Mahachai V, Suwangool P, Poovorawan Y. Gender difference in clinicopathologic features and survival of patients with hepatocellular carcinoma. World J Gastroenterol 2004;10:1547-50.

[43]   Nagasue N, Ono T, Yamanoi A, *et al*. Prognostic factors and survival after hepatic resection for hepatocellular carcinoma without cirrhosis. Br J Surg 2001;88:515-22.

[44]   Cong WM, Wu MC, Zhang XH, *et al*. Primary hepatocellular carcinoma in women of mainland China. A clinicopathologic analysis of 104 patients. Cancer 1993;71:2941-5.

[45]   Dohmen K, Shigematsu H, Irie K, Ishibashi H. Longer survival in female than male with hepatocellular carcinoma. J Gastroenterol Hepatol 2003;18:267-72.

[46]   Benvegnu L, Alberti A. Patterns of hepatocellular carcinoma development in hepatitis B virus and hepatitis C virus related cirrhosis. Antiviral Res 2001;52:199-207.

[47]   Farinati F, Sergio A, Giacomin A, *et al*. Is female sex a significant favorable prognostic factor in hepatocellular carcinoma? Eur J Gastroenterol Hepatol 2009;21:1212-8.

[48]   Lam CM, Yong JL, Chan AO, *et al*. Better survival in female patients with hepatocellular carcinoma: oral contraceptive pills related? J Clin Gastroenterol 2005;39:533-9.

[49]   Evans AA, Chen G, Ross EA, *et al*. Eight-year follow-up of the 90,000-person Haimen City cohort: I. Hepatocellular carcinoma mortality, risk factors, and gender differences. Cancer Epidemiol Biomarkers Prev 2002;11:369-76.

[50]   Nagasue N, Galizia G, Yukaya H, *et al*. Better survival in women than in men after radical resection of hepatocellular carcinoma. Hepatogastroenterology 1989;36:379-83.

[51]   Lee CC, Chau GY, Lui WY, *et al*. Better post-resectional survival in female cirrhotic patients with hepatocellular carcinoma. Hepatogastroenterology 2000;47:446-9.

[52]   Parkin DM, Srivatanakul P, Khlat M, *et al*. Liver cancer in Thailand. I. A case-control study of cholangiocarcinoma. Int J Cancer 1991;48:323-8.

[53]   Calvet X, Bruix J, Gines P, *et al*. Prognostic factors of hepatocellular carcinoma in the west: a multivariate analysis in 206 patients. Hepatology 1990;12:753-60.

[54]   Falkson G, Cnaan A, Schutt AJ, *et al*. Prognostic factors for survival in hepatocellular carcinoma. Cancer Res 1988;48:7314-8.

[55]   Lai CL, Gregory PB, Wu PC, *et al*. Hepatocellular carcinoma in Chinese males and females. Possible causes for the male predominance. Cancer 1987;60:1107-10.

[56] Chen WT, Chau GY, Lui WY, *et al.* Recurrent hepatocellular carcinoma after hepatic resection: prognostic factors and long-term outcome. Eur J Surg Oncol 2004;30:414-20.

[57] Poon RT, Fan ST. Evaluation of the new AJCC/UICC staging system for hepatocellular carcinoma after hepatic resection in Chinese patients. Surg Oncol Clin N Am 2003;12:35-50, viii.

[58] Wang J, Xu LB, Liu C, *et al.* Prognostic factors and outcome of 438 chinese patients with hepatocellular carcinoma underwent partial hepatectomy in a single center. World J Surg 2010;34:2434-41.

[59] Huang J, Li BK, Chen GH, *et al.* Long-term outcomes and prognostic factors of elderly patients with hepatocellular carcinoma undergoing hepatectomy. J Gastrointest Surg 2009;13:1627-35.

[60] Akashi Y, Koreeda C, Enomoto S, *et al.* Prognosis of unresectable hepatocellular carcinoma: an evaluation based on multivariate analysis of 90 cases. Hepatology 1991;14:262-8.

[61] Pawarode A, Tangkijvanich P, Voravud N. Outcomes of primary hepatocellular carcinoma treatment: an 8-year experience with 368 patients in Thailand. J Gastroenterol Hepatol 2000;15:860-4.

[62] Bruix J, Llovet JM. Major achievements in hepatocellular carcinoma. Lancet 2009;373:614-6.

CHAPTER 3

Body Iron and Chronic Liver Diseases

Ichiro Shimizu[1]*, Tomomi Matsumoto[2], Nozomi Suzuki[2], Chiaki Sagara[2], Yui Koizumi[2], Tsutoshi Asaki[1], Yoshiki Katakura[1] and Yosho Fukita[1]

[1]*Department of Gastroenterology and* [2]*Support Center for Medical Sciences, Seirei Yokohama Hospital, 215 Iwai-cho, Hodogaya-ku, Kanagawa 240-8521, Japan*

Abstract: As a target organ, the liver is particularly susceptible to excess iron levels. Hepatic iron overload induces mitochondrial injury and DNA mutagenesis, being an independent factor associated with hepatic fibrosis along with cell death, and increasing the risk of hepatocellular carcinoma development. In humans with iron overload due to either genetic or acquired causes, fibrosis and cirrhosis are hallmarks of liver disease. The clinical expression of genetic hemochromatosis is 5 to 10 times more frequent in men than in women, especially because of iron losses in women by menstruation and pregnancy. Iron deficiency is prevalent in females of reproductive age. Iron deficiency anemia is more commonly found in females than males. Women, especially before menopause, have lower iron stores in the liver. Hepcidin is a circulatory peptide synthesized in the liver that appears to regulate iron absorption in the duodenum. It is noteworthy that female mice express higher hepcidin levels in the liver than males, although it is not known whether women and men differ in the level of hepatic hepcidin expression. Sex-related differences in body iron storage and metabolism may be a potential candidate to explain in part the observed sex-related differences in many chronic liver diseases.

Keywords: Hepatic iron, iron overload, mitochondrial injury, hepatic fibrosis, oxidative stress, DNA mutagenesis, cell death, hemochromatosis, menstruation, pregnancy, iron deficiency anemia, hepcidin.

1. INTRODUCTION

Iron is an essential nutrient required for a variety of biochemical processes. It is a vital component of the heme in hemoglobin of red blood cells, myoglobin and cytochromes, and is also an essential cofactor for non-heme enzymes such as ribonucleotide reductase, the limiting enzyme for DNA synthesis [1]. The average daily dietary iron intake of an adult person is approximately 11-15 mg, and 6-12% of that amount (nearly 1 mg per day) is absorbed (Fig. **1**). Adults have a total of 3-5 g of iron. Approximately 65-75% is found in the heme. The liver stores 10-20% in the form of ferritin, which can be mobilized easily when needed. About 3-4% of the body's iron is in heme-bound myoglobin in striated muscle. Under physiological conditions, about 25 mg of iron per day is consumed by immature red blood cells in bone marrow for heme biosynthesis. The rest is distributed in other tissues [1]. There is no regulated pathway for the excretion of iron in the body except by blood loss or desquamated intestinal cells. The amount of iron loss is nearly 1 mg per day. When in excess iron is toxic because it produces reactive oxygen species (ROS) such as hydroxyl radicals that react readily with biological molecules, including proteins, lipids and DNA, leading to cell death and DNA mutagenesis [2]. As a target organ, the liver is particularly susceptible to excess iron levels.

2. LIVER PLAYS A MAJOR ROLE IN IRON HOMEOSTASIS IN THE BODY

Iron uptake and transport is tightly controlled. Liver plays an important role in iron homeostasis in the body, while liver is particularly susceptible to excess iron levels. Hepcidin, a circulatory antimicrobial peptide synthesized by the liver, regulates iron homeostasis by inhibiting the uptake of dietary iron in the duodenum and the export of iron from reticuloendothelial cells.

Unlike humans or rats, mice have 2 hepcidin genes, hepcidin1 and hepcidin2. The C-terminal 25 amino

*Address correspondence to Ichiro Shimizu: Department of Gastroenterology, Seirei Yokohama Hospital, 215 Iwai-cho, Hodogaya-ku, Yokohama, Kanagawa 240-8521, Japan; Tel: +81-45-715-3111; Fax: +81-45-715-3387; E-mail: ichiro.shimizu@showaclinic.jp

acid mature peptide region of mouse hepcidin1 shares higher homology with human hepcidin than mouse hepcidin2. Targeted disruption of hepcidin1 gene results in severe iron overload, demonstrating increased blood iron and ferritin levels as compared with controls [3], whereas mice overexpressing hepcidin1, but not hepcidin2, display anemia [4]. These data suggest a role for hepcidin1 but not hepcidin2 in the regulation of iron metabolism. It is noteworthy that female mice express higher levels of both hepcidin1 and hepcidin2 in the liver than males [5]. An increase in hepcidin levels would lead to a decrease in duodenal iron absorption and the mobilization of reticuloendothelial iron stores. This is achieved by hepcidin binding to the iron exporter, ferroportin, and inducing its internalization and degradation. It is not known whether female and male persons differ in the level of human hepcidin expression in the liver.

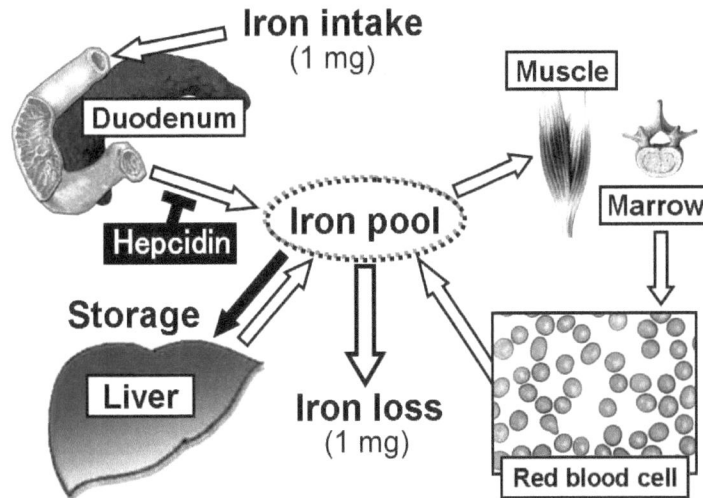

Fig. 1. Liver plays a major role in iron homeostasis in the body. Both the iron amount of uptake in the duodenum and loss by blood loss and desquamated intestinal cells are about 1 mg per day. Hepcidin, a circulatory peptide synthesized by the liver, regulates iron homeostasis by inhibiting the uptake of dietary iron in the duodenum.

3. FEMALES AND LOW IRON STORES IN THE LIVER

Iron deficiency is prevalent in females of reproductive age mainly due to the physiological loss of blood by menstruation and pregnancy throughout the world. Based on the differences between the amount of iron available for absorption and the increased requirement for iron, most females before menopause do not have adequate iron stores. Females experience iron deficiency anemia more commonly than males [6].

In the absence of hepatic inflammation, blood ferritin is a reliable marker of iron stores in the liver. In a study from Japan, blood ferritin levels were examined by sex and age in healthy individuals [7] (Fig. **2**). In males, the blood ferritin values reached the maximum level in the age group of 40 to 49 years and declined thereafter. By contrast, in females the blood ferritin remained relatively low until menopause, at a level which was one-fifth of that for males of comparable age, and reached the maximum level after menopause to approximately one-half of that for males of comparable age. These data correlate with the data obtained from the third National Health and Nutrition Examination Survey (NHANES III) in the United States [8], and indicate that females, especially before menopause, have lower iron stores in the liver.

Oxidative stress induced by hepatitis C virus (HCV) proteins and alcohol is suggested to be one of the mechanisms responsible for the down-regulation of hepcidin expression [9,10]. Ethanol produces ROS *via* the alcohol dehydrogenase (ADH)- and cytochrome P450 2E1 (CYP2E1)-metabolizing system. In addition, inflammation is a dominant and robust inducer of hepcidin gene transcription regardless of body iron levels [1]. Interleukin-6 (IL-6) and possibly other proinflammatory cytokines such as interleukin-1 (IL-1) are the major players in this process. Estradiol is a strong endogenous antioxidant that inhibits ROS production processes and stimulates antioxidant enzyme activities [11,12]. There is a large body of evidence indicating that the decline in ovarian function with menopause is associated with spontaneous increase in proinflammatory cytokines, tumor necrosis factor-α (TNF-α), IL-1 and IL-6 [13]. Estradiol, at physiological concentrations, inhibits the spontaneous secretion of proinflammatory cytokines in murine peritoneal macrophages [14] and human peripheral blood mononuclear cells [15,16]. Furthermore, male mice display lower hepcidin expression compared to female mice following treatment with ethanol [9]. The more pronounced down-regulation of hepcidin among males is abrogated by antioxidants. In a preliminary report, concomitant administration of estradiol resulted in a reduction in blood levels of liver enzyme (ALT) and ferritin and hepatic iron stores in a young male patient with chronic hepatitis C and irradiation-induced testicular dysfunction, in whom testosterone replacement therapy was initiated at puberty [17]. Taken together, these data suggest that, besides iron, hepcidin may be also regulated by female sex-specific factors including estrogens.

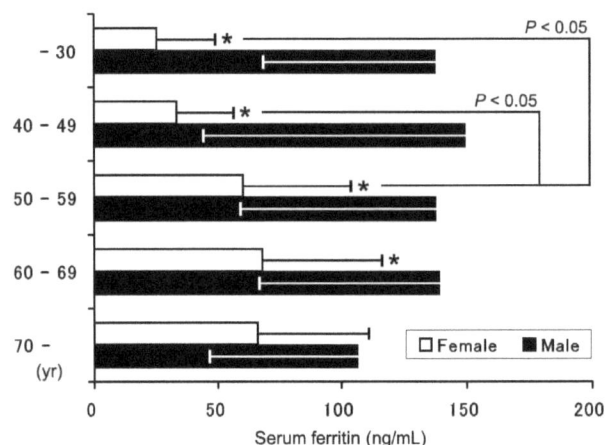

Fig. 2. Age-specific blood ferritin levels among females and males in 305 healthy Japanese individuals (mean age 50.6 years, 52.8% females) [7]. Blood ferritin levels reflect the iron stores in the liver. Premenopausal females have a one-fifth level of the blood ferritin for males of comparable age. $*P < 0.05$ compared with males of comparable age.

4. HEPATIC IRON OVERLOAD

An analysis of the NHANES III data in the United States showed that patients with chronic hepatitis C have higher blood levels of iron and ferritin compared to healthy subjects [18]. The lobular and cellular distributions of the stainable iron in the liver of chronic hepatitis C patients are correlated with hepatitis severity [19], although most patients with chronic hepatitis C do not have an elevated hepatic iron concentration despite the abnormal blood iron parameters [20].

In a clinical study with liver biopsies from sex- and age- matched untreated patients with chronic hepatitis B (n=20) and chronic hepatitis C (n=43), the hepatocyte iron-staining score is similar in patients with chronic hepatitis B and C groups [21]. The frequencies of iron-staining in chronic hepatitis B and C are greater than the iron-staining frequency in alcoholic liver disease [22]. Hepatic iron overload is an independent factor associated with hepatic fibrosis along with cell death [23]. Stainable iron in non-cancerous and cancerous liver specimens in Chinese patients with hepatitis B virus (HBV)-associated hepatocellular carcinoma (HCC) is preferentially enriched in hepatocytes replicating HBV [24]. Genetic hemochromatosis, a prevalent iron overload disorder among the Caucasian population, is the abnormalities of genes such as *HFE* [25]. The clinical expression of genetic hemochromatosis is 5 to 10 times more frequent in males than in females. Male patients with genetic hemochromatosis accumulate more iron and have a higher incidence of the liver injury [26]. In males with genetic hemochromatosis complicated with HCC, hepatitis B surface antigen (HBsAg) seropositivity is higher (6.2%) than in male blood donors from sex- and age-matched control groups (0.075%), whereas 0.04% of female controls have HBsAg seropositivity and the female patients with and without HCC show no blood HBV marker [27]. Moreover, iron reduction therapy by repeated phlebotomy improves hepatocyte injury in patients with HCV infection [28]. Phlebotomy is the opening of a vein to remove blood. These data suggest that hepatic iron overload may facilitate viral replication in hepatocytes, or hepatocytes containing virus may tend to accumulate iron.

It is widely recognized that hepatic iron overload develops in a significant portion of individuals who consume alcohol on a chronic basis. Chronic alcohol consumption in moderate to excess quantities results in increased blood ferritin, which may thus result in increased hepatic iron stores [29]. Females drink less alcohol and have fewer alcohol-related problems than males [30]. The data demonstrate that chronic alcohol consumption-related hepatic iron stores are less likely in females than in males.

There is growing concern in clinical practice with regard to the development of non-alcoholic fatty liver disease (NAFLD). Its name implies a histological picture that is indistinguishable from alcoholic liver disease. Although in most cases, fatty liver does not progress to more severe liver disease, approximately 15-20% of patients have histological signs of hepatic fibrosis and necroinflammation, indicating the presence of non-alcoholic steatohepatitis (NASH). These patients are at a higher risk of developing cirrhosis and HCC [31]. NAFLD is more prevalent in males, and there is a male predominance for NASH as well [32]. The pathogenesis of NAFLD and NASH is associated with insulin resistance and metabolic syndrome *via* oxidative stress and inflammation [33]. Although the data regarding actual hepatic iron overload in HAFLD has been somewhat conflicting, NASH patients have increased hepatic iron accumulation [34,35].

5. CONCLUSION

Margaret Thatcher became the first woman prime minister of the United Kingdom in 1979, and the longest-serving in the 20th century to win three consecutive elections. A highly respected world leader renowned for her tough leadership style, Thatcher earned the title "the Iron Lady." In fact, however, Thatcher was not a lady of "the iron" biologically. The reason is because there was not excessive iron in her tough liver. As a target organ, the liver is particularly susceptible to excess iron levels. Females have less total body storage iron and lower iron stores in the liver, possibly because of iron loss during menstruation and increased requirements during pregnancy. Sex-related differences in body iron storage and metabolism may be a potential candidate to explain in part the observed sex-related differences in many chronic liver diseases. The lower hepatic iron stores provide help to females by protecting the liver against chronic liver injury. It would be better for females never to have a real "iron" liver. Ms, you can never become an "iron lady."

REFERENCES

[1]   Zhang AS, Enns CA. Iron homeostasis: recently identified proteins provide insight into novel control mechanisms. J Biol Chem 2009;284:711-5.
[2]   Berger M, de Hazen M, Nejjari A, *et al.* Radical oxidation reactions of the purine moiety of 2'-deoxyribonucleosides and DNA by iron-containing minerals. Carcinogenesis 1993;14:41-6.
[3]   Lesbordes-Brion JC, Viatte L, Bennoun M, *et al.* Targeted disruption of the hepcidin 1 gene results in severe hemochromatosis. Blood 2006;108:1402-5.
[4]   Lou DQ, Nicolas G, Lesbordes JC, *et al.* Functional differences between hepcidin 1 and 2 in transgenic mice. Blood 2004;103:2816-21.
[5]   Courselaud B, Troadec MB, Fruchon S, *et al.* Strain and gender modulate hepatic hepcidin 1 and 2 mRNA expression in mice. Blood Cells Mol Dis 2004;32:283-9.
[6]   Looker AC, Dallman PR, Carroll MD, *et al.* Prevalence of iron deficiency in the United States. JAMA 1997;277:973-6.
[7]   Shimizu I, Kohno N, Tamaki K, *et al.* Female hepatology: favorable role of estrogen in chronic liver disease with hepatitis B virus infection. World J Gastroenterol 2007;13:4295-305.
[8]   Zacharski LR, Ornstein DL, Woloshin S, Schwartz LM. Association of age, sex, and race with body iron stores in adults: analysis of NHANES III data. Am Heart J 2000;140:98-104.
[9]   Harrison-Findik DD, Schafer D, Klein E, *et al.* Alcohol metabolism-mediated oxidative stress down-regulates hepcidin transcription and leads to increased duodenal iron transporter expression. J Biol Chem 2006;281:22974-82.
[10]   Nishina S, Hino K, Korenaga M, *et al.* Hepatitis C virus-induced reactive oxygen species raise hepatic iron level in mice by reducing hepcidin transcription. Gastroenterology 2008;134:226-38.
[11]   Lu G, Shimizu I, Cui X, *et al.* Antioxidant and antiapoptotic activities of idoxifene and estradiol in hepatic fibrosis in rats. Life Sci 2004;74:897-907.

[12]   Itagaki T, Shimizu I, Cheng X, *et al.* Opposing effects of oestradiol and progesterone on intracellular pathways and activation processes in the oxidative stress induced activation of cultured rat hepatic stellate cells. Gut 2005;54:1782-9.

[13]   Pfeilschifter J, Koditz R, Pfohl M, Schatz H. Changes in Proinflammatory Cytokine Activity after Menopause. Endocr Rev 2002;23:90-119.

[14]   Huang H, He J, Yuan Y, *et al.* Opposing effects of estradiol and progesterone on the oxidative stress-induced production of chemokine and proinflammatory cytokines in murine peritoneal macrophages. J Med Invest 2008;55:133-41.

[15]   Rachon D, Mysliwska J, Suchecka-Rachon K, *et al.* Effects of oestrogen deprivation on interleukin-6 production by peripheral blood mononuclear cells of postmenopausal women. J Endocrinol 2002;172:387-95.

[16]   Yuan Y, Shimizu I, Shen M, *et al.* Effects of estradiol and progesterone on the proinflammatory cytokine production by mononuclear cells from patients with chronic hepatitis C. World J Gastroenterol 2008;14:2200-7.

[17]   Shimizu I, Omoya T, Kondo Y, *et al.* Estrogen therapy in a male patient with chronic hepatitis C and irradiation-induced testicular dysfunction. Intern Med 2001;40:100-4.

[18]   Shan Y, Lambrecht RW, Bonkovsky HL. Association of hepatitis C virus infection with serum iron status: analysis of data from the third National Health and Nutrition Examination Survey. Clin Infect Dis 2005;40:834-41.

[19]   Barton AL, Banner BF, Cable EE, Bonkovsky HL. Distribution of iron in the liver predicts the response of chronic hepatitis C infection to interferon therapy. Am J Clin Pathol 1995;103:419-24.

[20]   Arber N, Konikoff FM, Moshkowitz M, *et al.* Increased serum iron and iron saturation without liver iron accumulation distinguish chronic hepatitis C from other chronic liver diseases. Dig Dis Sci 1994;39:2656-9.

[21]   Mohammad Alizadeh AH, Fallahian F, Alavian SM, *et al.* Insulin resistance in chronic hepatitis B and C. Indian J Gastroenterol 2006;25:286-9.

[22]   Kaji K, Nakanuma Y, Sasaki M, *et al.* Hemosiderin deposition in portal endothelial cells: a novel hepatic hemosiderosis frequent in chronic viral hepatitis B and C. Hum Pathol 1995;26:1080-5.

[23]   Rigamonti C, Andorno S, Maduli E, *et al.* Gender and liver fibrosis in chronic hepatitis: the role of iron status. Aliment Pharmacol Ther 2005;21:1445-51.

[24]   Zhou XD, DeTolla L, Custer RP, London WT. Iron, ferritin, hepatitis B surface and core antigens in the livers of Chinese patients with hepatocellular carcinoma. Cancer 1987;59:1430-7.

[25]   Eijkelkamp EJ, Yapp TR, Powell LW. HFE-associated hereditary hemochromatosis. Can J Gastroenterol 2000;14:121-5.

[26]   Siemons LJ, Mahler CH. Hypogonadotropic hypogonadism in hemochromatosis: recovery of reproductive function after iron depletion. J Clin Endocrinol Metab 1987;65:585-7.

[27]   Deugnier Y, Battistelli D, Jouanolle H, *et al.* Hepatitis B virus infection markers in genetic haemochromatosis. A study of 272 patients. J Hepatol 1991;13:286-90.

[28]   Yano M, Hayashi H, Yoshioka K, *et al.* A significant reduction in serum alanine aminotransferase levels after 3-month iron reduction therapy for chronic hepatitis C: a multicenter, prospective, randomized, controlled trial in Japan. J Gastroenterol 2004;39:570-4.

[29]   Rouault TA. Hepatic iron overload in alcoholic liver disease: why does it occur and what is its role in pathogenesis? Alcohol 2003;30:103-6.

[30]   Nolen-Hoeksema S. Gender differences in risk factors and consequences for alcohol use and problems. Clin Psychol Rev 2004;24:981-1010.

[31]   Harrison SA, Kadakia S, Lang KA, Schenker S. Nonalcoholic steatohepatitis: what we know in the new millennium. Am J Gastroenterol 2002;97:2714-24.

[32]   Clark JM, Brancati FL, Diehl AM. Nonalcoholic fatty liver disease. Gastroenterology 2002;122:1649-57.

[33]   Cortez-Pinto H, de Moura MC, Day CP. Non-alcoholic steatohepatitis: from cell biology to clinical practice. J Hepatol 2006;44:197-208.

[34]   George DK, Goldwurm S, MacDonald GA, *et al.* Increased hepatic iron concentration in nonalcoholic steatohepatitis is associated with increased fibrosis. Gastroenterology 1998;114:311-8.

[35]   Bonkovsky HL, Jawaid Q, Tortorelli K, *et al.* Non-alcoholic steatohepatitis and iron: increased prevalence of mutations of the HFE gene in non-alcoholic steatohepatitis. J Hepatol 1999;31:421-9.

CHAPTER 4

HCV Carriers With Normal Alanine Aminotransferase Levels

Claudio Puoti*

Department of Internal Medicine, Gastroenterology and Liver Unit, Marino General Hospital, Rome, ITALY

Abstract: Approximately 30% of patients with chronic hepatitis C virus (HCV) infection show persistently normal alanine aminotransferase (ALT) levels. Although formerly referred to as 'healthy' or 'asymptomatic' HCV carriers, and thus historically excluded from antiviral treatment, it has now become clear that the majority of these patients have some degree of histological liver damage.

Although liver disease is usually minimal/mild and fibrosis is generally absent or minimal, the natural history of HCV carriers with persistently normal ALT levels (PNALT) is probably not always so benign, and the possibility of a more severe evolution of liver disease among patients with PNALT cannot be ruled out. Several studies reported a significant progression of fibrosis in approximately 20-30% of the patients with well-defined ALT normality, and the development of hepatocellular carcinoma in some cases has been described, despite persistent ALT normality. Sudden worsening of disease with ALT increase and histological deterioration has been described after up to 15 years of follow-up.

Recent studies have shown that combined antiviral treatment with pegylated interferon plus ribavirin might allow a sustained virological response in up to 70-80% of patients harboring HCV type 2 or 3, and approximately 50% of those infected with genotype 1. Thus, the advent of these new therapeutic options has shifted treatment targets toward eradication of underlying infection, with therapy decision based on age, severity of disease and likelihood of response rather than on aminotransferase levels.

Keywords: Alanine aminotransferase, carrier, cirrhosis, fibrosis, HCV, Hhpatitis, healthy, interferon, normal, ribavirin, virological response.

1. INTRODUCTION

Infection with hepatitis C virus (HCV) is a major cause of chronic hepatitis, cirrhosis, end-stage liver disease and hepatocellular carcinoma (HCC) [1-3]. Chronic HCV infection is associated with elevation of serum alanine aminotransferase (ALT) activity in many patients; however, up to 30% of patients with chronic HCV infection show persistently normal ALT levels (PNALT), and another 40% have minimally raised ALT values [3-5].

Although formerly considered as 'healthy' or 'asymptomatic' HCV carriers [6], it has now become clear that the majority of these patients have some degree of histological liver damage [6-11].

Thus, it is time to challenge the early opinions that:

a)   Chronic HCV infection with normal ALT levels does always mean a benign and healthy state [12],

b)   The rate of disease progression and the severity of liver damage are invariably lower than in patients with elevated ALT [13], and

c)   These people should be monitored but not treated [14].

Despite a lot of papers and data, several controversies still exist regarding the concept of *"normal"* ALT levels, the definition of *"persistently"* normal ALT values, the demographic, virological and histological features of these subjects, the natural history of *"biochemically silent"* HCV chronic infection, and the need for antiviral treatment in this subset of patients [15, 16].

*Address correspondence to Claudio Puoti: Claudio Puoti, Department of Internal Medicine, Marino General Hospital, *Via* XXIV Maggio, 00047 Marino, Rome, Italy; Tel: 0039 6 9327 7681; Fax 0039 6 9327 3043; E-mail: puoti@epatologia.org

Ichiro Shimizu (Ed)

In this chapter, we would examine the main open issues in the management of these so-called "healthy" subjects, chronically carrying the Hepatitis C Virus.

2. TERMINOLOGY AND DEFINITIONS

The criteria for the diagnosis of HCV carriers with normal aminotransferases have been proposed by the first NIH Consensus Development Conference "Management of Hepatitis C" in 1997 [13] and revised during the "EASL Consensus Conference on Hepatitis C" in 1999 [14]. On the basis of these criteria, the diagnosis of HCV carriers with normal aminotransferase values can be made in the presence of:

     a)   Positivity of anti-HCV antibodies.

     b)   Positivity of HCV RNA by RT-PCR.

     c)   Normal ALT levels in at least three tests carried out at least two months apart, over a period of six months.

Several definitions have been used worldwide to identify subjects with chronic HCV infection, but normal aminotransferase levels, such as:

     a)   Healthy HCV carrier.

     b)   Biochemically silent HCV carrier.

     c)   Asymptomatic HCV carrier hepatitis C.

     d)   HCV carrier with PNALT.

The definition 'HCV healthy carrier', albeit of widespread use, should be avoided as only a very small part of carriers with normal aminotransferase levels have normal liver histology.

The definition 'biochemically silent HCV carrier' has been used by some authors with reference to a normal liver biochemistry. Although appropriate, this definition is not currently adopted all over the world.

The definition 'asymptomatic HCV carrier' is commonly used. It is, however, an improper definition, since the aminotransferase levels cannot be considered a symptom.

'HCV carrier with PNALT is the most accurate definition, and the one which should be universally adopted [17].

3. AMINOTRANSFERASE ACTIVITY AND THE CHRONIC HCV CARRIER STATE

It is well known that ALT is located in the liver tissue, leaking into the systemic circulation as a consequence of hepatocellular injury of various severity. Consequently, serum ALT determination is widely used for the diagnosis and follow up of patients with chronic hepatitis C [18].

However, it is now accepted that scarce correlation does exist between serum ALT levels and the degree of liver damage and fibrosis, evaluated through liver biopsy or non-invasive tools [19]. This finding might be explained by whether liver cell death occurs mainly *via* apoptosis and/or necrosis [18].

Therefore, as only a weak correlation exists between serum ALT and the severity of liver damage, ALT measurement provides no differentiation of reversible vs. irreversible damage [20]. Moreover, although it is a good marker of liver cell necroinflammation, ALT activity is not directly related to fibrosis. There may be reduced serum ALT levels in cirrhosis in which liver function is abnormal, and conversely increased ALT in benign acute injury (*e.g.*, HAV hepatitis) when liver function may be normal.

Current upper limits for ALT were set, on average, at 40 U/L (within a range of 30-50 U/L) in studies on HCV carriers conducted over the past 20 years. Such thresholds, however, were mostly computed in the

1980s, when ALT testing was introduced as a surrogate marker for the screening of non-A and non-B hepatitis among blood donors and before anti-HCV testing and restrictive behavioral criteria were implemented [21]. Furthermore, the so-called "reference" populations were likely to include substantial proportions of individuals with nonalcoholic fatty liver disease (NAFLD), now recognized as the most prevalent cause of chronic liver disease in developed countries. In this regard, several studies suggest that the current reference ranges for ALT normal values used in clinical practice underestimate the actual frequency of chronic liver disease [22, 23]. Furthermore, the ALT reference ranges currently used in clinical practice underevaluate the actual frequency of liver disease in this subset of patients; indeed, current evidence suggests that existing "normal" ALT thresholds are too high [17] and should be lowered by 25-30%, thus setting the "optimal" ALT threshold at 30 U/L for males and 20 U/L for females [21].

Furthermore, the distribution of ALT values in the general population is strongly influenced by extra hepatic factors including gender, ethnicity, blood groups and obesity [21].

4. "REPEATEDLY" NORMAL OR "PERSISTENTLY" NORMAL ALT LEVELS?

Characterization of histological features and disease progression in individuals with HCV and normal ALT is complicated by the definitions applied to select patients [17]. There is relevant disparity between studies according to the definition of ALT normal range and of *persistent* normality; furthermore, great variability exists in selection criteria, leading to inclusion of patients with fluctuating ALT, PNALT and near-normal ALT.

As above underlined, former Consensus Conferences [5, 13, 14] suggested that the definition of HCV carriers with PNALT should be made on the basis of at least three normal ALT values 2 months apart over a 6-month period. However, this is a too short observation period, as in clinical practice sudden increases in ALT levels are not uncommon, even at interval longer than 6 months [24]. Several studies [7, 25] have shown that many subjects referred to as HCV carriers with PNALT on the basis of this definition could have ALT flare-ups during the follow-up, thus proving that even prolonged observation periods might be not adequate to distinguish patients with persistent or transient ALT normality. These flares have been in particular observed among HCV-2 infected patients [26].

It is known that during the course of HCV infection ALT levels could fluctuate, with long periods of biochemical remission [17]. It has been suggested that at least two different subsets of HCV carriers exist: patients with wide temporal ALT fluctuations, that could be within the normal range for several months, and true 'biochemically silent' carriers, showing persistently normal ALT values [4]. It is not known whether these subgroups have different natural history and disease progression [6]. Liver histological activity has been found to be more severe among carriers with ALT flares than in those with persistently normal ALT levels [25].

Thus the observation period should not be shorter than 12-18 months, and ALT determinations should be performed every 2-3 months [15]. Indeed, *repeatedly* normal does not necessarily mean *persistently* normal [4].

5. EPIDEMIOLOGICAL FEATURES

Most HCV carriers are discovered after blood donation, screening of family members of anti-HCV positive subjects, case finding in high risk groups, extra hepatic manifestations (cryoglobulinaemia, lymphoma), or medical check-ups [17].

Three different scenarios might be seen: a) a patient who has just been found anti-HCV with "normal" ALT (sporadic determinations); b) A patient who has been referred as anti-HCV with "normal" ALT on 1 or more occasions in the last 6 months, and c) a patient known to have been anti-HCV with "normal" ALT for a long period of time.

The overall prevalence of HCV carriers with normal ALT values has been estimated between 1.5% and 12%, in Italian population-based surveys [27-29], with a strong geographic prevalence gradient. In a study performed in a population of in-patients with normal ALT admitted to a General Hospital because of non hepatic diseases, this prevalence was found to be 4% [30].

In a number of studies, the demographic characteristics of HCV carriers with normal ALT levels have been described and compared with those of HCV patients with biochemical evidence of chronic liver disease. Overall, data from the literature indicate a prevalence of females, from 58% to 90% in the different studies [1-8, 31-36]. Discordant results have been reported with regards to risk of transmitting HCV infection among sexual partners and household contacts [37, 38].

For these patients, the recommendations to limit viral transmission (in relation to sexual intercourse, pregnancy, breast feeding, intrafamilial spreading) are not different from those indicated for patients with increased ALT levels [1, 2, 5, 17].

6. VIROLOGICAL ASPECTS

Several studies have examined the virological characteristics of HCV carriers with normal aminotransferases, with conflicting results.

6.1. HCV Genotype

Italian studies [8, 39, 40] reported a higher prevalence of genotype 2 in carriers with normal ALT values and of genotype 1b in patients with increased ALT values. Conversely, studies carried out in U.S.A. [33] and Japan [41] reported a higher prevalence of genotype 1b in carriers with normal aminotransferase values. These discrepancies can be attributed to differences in the selection criteria, to a different geographical distribution of genotypes and to the differences in the prevalence of drug addicts in the study populations [17].

No clear-cut correlation has been found between genotype and severity of the histological lesions [25, 39, 40, 42].

6.2. Quantitative Viremia and Viral Quasispecies

No significant differences exist in HCV RNA serum levels between patients with PNALT and those with abnormal ALT levels [1-4]. Furthermore, no correlations exist between the entity of serum HCV load and the presence or severity of histological liver disease [1, 2, 43, 44]. Thus, HCV RNA levels do not predict the risk or severity of ALT flares during the follow-up [43].

By consequence, it has been stated that HCV RNA testing using a quantitative assay and HCV genotyping should be determined only in patients for whom antiviral treatment is being considered, in order to determine the duration of treatment and the likelihood of response. In other cases, the evaluation of serum viral load is not necessary and thus expensive and unhelpful [1, 2, 17, 43].

Several studies did address the significance and the role of quasi species in carriers with PNALT. Some authors [41] reported no differences in the viral quasispecies between subjects with normal ALT levels and patients with increased aminotransferases, while others [45] reported a greater incidence of HVR1 changes in carriers with persistently normal aminotransferase values. It has been reported [46] that the core region was highly conserved in carriers with normal ALT levels, as compared to those with abnormal liver enzymes.

In conclusion, the HCV carrier with normal ALT levels does not have a specific "virological profile" and no definite relationships have been found between genotype, levels of viremia, quasispecies, and severity or progression of liver disease.

7. LIVER HISTOLOGY

Despite early opinion that HCV carriers with PNALT should be considered as *healthy* people, thus invariably showing normal liver, it has now become clear that "normal" does not always mean "healthy"

[4]. Indeed, it has been clearly showed that the majority of HCV carriers with PNALT have some degree of liver damage on liver biopsy [5-12]. Liver disease is usually minimal/mild and fibrosis is generally absent or minimal [1-12, 47, 48]. Overall, the extent of necroinflammation and fibrosis is generally lower in patients with normal ALT compared to those with elevated ALT [1-4, 17]. Shiffman *et al.* [36] found that patients with normal ALT levels had significantly lower inflammation and fibrosis scores on liver biopsy examination than patients with elevated ALT levels, but almost two-thirds had portal fibrosis and 10% had bridging fibrosis. A multicentric study from Italy [25] found normal liver in less than 17% of patients with PNALT, minimal or mild chronic hepatitis occurring in up to 78% of the cases and severe CH or cirrhosis in 5 %.

Several studies comparing liver histology in HCV patients with normal or elevated ALT levels have reported equivalent liver damage in the two patient populations [49-52], while others found that in persons with PNALT progression of fibrosis was less pronounced than in those with abnormal ALT levels, thus suggesting that patients with normal ALT and mild histology can safely defer treatment [53].

In summary, the majority of available studies indicate that not all HCV carriers have mild liver disease [4, 7, 18-20, 26, 31-36, 54, 55]. Cirrhosis has been reported with varying incidence (1.5%-14%), and case reports of HCC despite persistent ALT normality have also been published [56-59]. No correlation between baseline ALT activity, HCV RNA level, and liver histology was observed in patients with normal ALT levels.

Again, the high variability in the prevalence and severity of the histological abnormalities found in different studies may be attributable, at least in part, to the number of patients assessed or to the application of different definitions of normal serum ALT levels [1-4].

8. NATURAL HISTORY

The natural history of HCV carriers with PNALT is probably not always benign, and the possibility of a more severe evolution of liver disease in this subset of patients cannot be ruled out. Spontaneous resolution of HCV infection has been reported rarely in patients with normal ALT (less than 15% after 5-7 years of follow up) [56].

Several studies showed a significant progression of fibrosis in approximately 20-30% of the patients with well-defined ALT normality [12, 44, 48, 49, 56]. Sudden worsening of disease with ALT increase and histological deterioration has been described after up to 15 years of follow-up [10, 26, 49].

A prospective Italian study [47] evaluated 25 subjects maintaining persistently normal ALT values for a total follow-up of 5 years. Liver biopsies carried out at the beginning and at the end of the observation period, showed that the scores for necroinflammatory activity and fibrosis remained unchanged. Other authors reported the spontaneous elimination of viremia in 15% of their patients after 3-7 years of observation [56]. In the study by Martinot-Peignoux *et al.* [7] both the activity and fibrosis remained unchanged at the second biopsy carried out in 24 patients after an average follow-up of 3.5 years.

Hui *et al.* [49] found that subjects with PNALT and an initial fibrosis of F0/F1 were less prone to develop progression of fibrosis than those with raised ALT levels, while the difference was not significant when patients with baseline F2 fibrosis were compared. Thus, the higher the severity of baseline liver damage, the faster the progression of the disease, despite biochemical normality.

Lawson *et al.* [54] found that fibrosis progression between paired biopsies was similar for patients with ALT levels persistently < 30 IU/L (0.33 ± 0.94 Ishak fibrosis points/year), ALT levels persistently < 40 IU/L (0.35 ± 0.82) and for those with elevated ALT (0.19 ± 0.48). The authors did conclude that the majority of those defined as PNALT patients subsequently have a similar risk of disease progression than patients with elevated ALT levels and, therefore, warrant the same consideration with regard to treatment.

No predictive factors for ALT flares have been identified [1-4], and elevations of ALT above normal occur independently of gender, baseline ALT, baseline HCV RNA and genotype [43].

However, a recent study suggests a greater risk of ALT flares (and a more rapid progression to fibrosis) in patients infected with genotype 2 compared with genotype 1 [26] although an influence of additional factors cannot be ruled out. For example, a high proportion of HCV-2 infected females with normal ALT frequently experience an increase in ALT levels during middle age, possibly due to hormones, obesity or a number of other cofactors. However, these patients may experience long periods of biochemical remission.

It is not clear why some carriers suffer from these sudden biochemical flares with subsequent histological worsening of the disease [4]. Several mechanisms have been suggested, such as virological features (genotype 2), steatosis of the liver, cofactors (HBV coinfection, alcohol abuse), BMI increase over time, late immune modifications, shift of apoptosis toward necrosis [15].

The appearance of HCC in subjects with PNALT has been suggested [56-58]. Some studies reported the occurrence of HCC in HCV carriers with PNALT but chronic liver damage [56, 57], while other authors did report the appearance of HCC in a patient with otherwhise "healthy" liver [58].

A paper from Japan [59] showed HCC occurrence in 9.8% of carriers with PNALT (48/519) during a 10 year follow up. The risk of HCC was higher in patients with high-normal ALT and platelet count < 150.000 than in those with persistently low-normal ALT and platelet count > 150.000.

9. SHOULD HCV CARRIERS WITH PNALT BE TREATED?

The earliest guidelines discouraged interferon (IFN) treatment in patients with PNALT outside of clinical trials [13, 14]. The main reasons for this statement were: a) most patients with chronic HCV infection and PNALT have low-grade liver fibrosis; b) they seem to be at low risk of disease progression; c) antiviral therapy is very expensive; d) there are several side effects of therapy, sometime severe, and e) response rates to IFN monotherapy were exceedingly low (<10-15%), with a risk of ALT flares in up to 50% of patients during treatment.

On the other hand, it has been stressed that these patients often have features traditionally associated with a good therapeutic response, such as mild histological lesions, prevalence of females and genotype non-1 infection [17]. Moreover, given the possibility of ALT flares during follow-up (which invariably accelerate the progression of fibrosis and worsen histological activity), the utility of deferring therapy has been questioned [1-3].

Conventional IFN α monotherapy has been evaluated in patients with persistently normal or near normal ALT levels (<1.5 ULN) [60-65]. The overall efficacy of IFN α was found to be very low, although not different than that seen in patients with elevated ALT, and sustained virological response (SVR) was attained by approximately 15-23% [17]. An ALT flare during the treatment or the follow-up has been reported in approximately 47% of patients, and has been attributed to enhanced immunity or cytotoxicity. The high incidence of ALT flares raised concerns regarding the risk of conventional IFN monotherapy compared with only modest benefit [1-3].

The introduction of the combination of Pegylated IFN (PEG-IFN) plus ribavirin (RBV) has led to overall response rates of more than 50%, with a favourable risk/benefit ratio even in patients with benign or slowly progressing disease.

The first multicentre, randomised study of PEG-IFN α 2a (180 μg weekly) plus RBV (800 mg daily) for 24 or 48 weeks in patients with PNALT found an overall sustained virological response (SVR) rate of 30% in those treated for 24 weeks and 52% in those treated for 48 weeks [66]. The response rates were 13% and 40% in patients with genotype 1b carriers and 72% and 78% in persons harbouring genotype 2 or 3.

The adverse reactions were no different from those observed in patients with abnormal ALT levels. The adverse event profile was typical of that expected, with no new events identified. Reported adverse events were generally mild in severity, the most common being headache, fatigue and myalgia, which were also noted in untreated controls. Transient, mild elevations in serum ALT (<60 U/L) were detected in 38% of treated patients and in 45% of controls [66].

It should also be stressed that ALT levels increased during the one-year follow-up period in more than 50% of the untreated PNALT patients in this placebo-controlled study.

However, in this study the subjects with HCV-1 were treated with a fixed RBV dose (800 mg/day) that is lower than that universally recommended for these patients (1000-1200 mg/day, depending on body weight), as the study was initiated before the optimal treatment regimen for these patients had been established. As a consequence of this, the reported response rate may be lower than it would be expected when the standard dose of RBV is used.

More recently, simulation studies [67] suggest that the SVR rates might significantly increase in HCV-1 patients when the standard weight-adjusted dose of RBV is administered. In these patients, the probability of SVR could increase almost linearly with RBV dose per kilogram of body weight. Other baseline factors predicted to increase the likelihood of SVR in both groups were younger age, lower HCV RNA level, Caucasian race, absence of cirrhosis and increasing ALT quotient. The analysis revealed that there are no consistent differences between genotype 1 patients with persistently normal or elevated ALT levels with respect to the influence of individual factors on predictions of SVR. In conclusion, this study showed that treatment of HCV genotype 1 patients with persistently normal ALT levels for 48 weeks with the currently recommended dose of RBV (1000 or 1200 mg/ day) in combination with PEG-IFN α 2a will result in SVR rates comparable to those achieved in patients with elevated ALT levels [67].

The efficacy and safety of antiviral treatment with PEG-IFN α 2a plus RBV were confirmed in clinical practice by a multicentric Italian study, enrolling 88 HCV carriers (53 females) with well-defined ALT normality [68]. This was the first study evaluating in real-life practice the efficacy of PEG-IFN plus RBV treatment of HCV carriers with PNALT using weight-adjusted RBV doses in HCV-1 patients.

36% of the patients in study did harbor HCV type 1, 52% genotype 2, and the remainder had genotype 3. 72 out of the patients had liver biopsy, while in the others transient hepatic elastography was performed. Normal histology was found in 19 % of the 72 patients undergoing biopsy, minimal fibrosis in 76%, F2-F3 fibrosis in 4 % and cirrhosis in 1%. Liver stiffness evaluated by hepatic elastography was normal (less than 7 kilopascal, kP) in 62% of the patients, mild (fibrosis F2-F3, 7 to 12 kPa) in 25% of the patients, and indicative of cirrhosis (>12 kPa) in 13% of the patients.

All the patients enrolled in this study received PEG-IFN α 2a 180 mg once weekly plus RBV 800 mg/day for 24 weeks (HCV-2 and -3), or 1000-1200 mg/day for 48 weeks (HCV-1). Rapid virological response (RVR) was seen in 66/88 patients (75%): 19/32 HCV-1 (59%), 40/46 HCV-2 (87%) and 7/10 HCV-3 patients. Younger patients, leaner subjects and patients with non-1 genotype or lower baseline HCV RNA levels were more likely to achieve an RVR. SVR was seen in 69/88 patients (78%): 20/32 HCV-1 patients (62%), 41/46 HCV-2 patients (89%) and 8/10 (80%) HCV-3 patients. The overall SVR rate was 88% in patients with RVR (58/66) and 50% in those without RVR [68].

Baseline viral load did not influence the rate of SVR in patients with HCV-2 and -3. In contrast, in patients with HCV-1, a relationship although not significant was seen between the rate of SVR and the baseline HCV RNA levels: SVR was seen in 11/12 patients (92%) with HCV RNA < 800 x 10^3 IU/ml and in 9/20 (45%) of those with HCV RNA serum levels > 800 x 10^3 IU/ml. The SVR rates were influenced by the gender of the patients: 76% of the patients showing SVR were females. By stratifying patients according to ALT values, no differences in SVR rates were seen between patients with "low-normal" ALT (ALT levels < 50% of the ULN) and those with "high-normal" ALT (ALT levels > 50% of the ULN). No ALT flares were seen during antiviral treatment. Side effects were not different from those seen among patients with abnormal ALT treated with the same schedules during the same period. No drop outs were observed. The appearance of anaemia was observed in 21 patients (24%), but reduction of RBV according to the protocol study was needed in only five patients, three of which failed to have SVR. No severe adverse events requiring dosage modifications or treatment premature withdrawal were reported. In particular, no signs or symptoms of thyroid dysfunction were seen.

The unusual high response rates seen in this study in patents with HCV-1 type was explained by the authors by the high prevalence of females, the mild degree of liver damage, the relatively low mean age and the normal BMI values observed in the majority of the patients in study.

The importance of RVR as a predictor of sustained viral clearance was further evaluated in a second study from the same Italian group [69]. It is known that RVR is now considered the strongest predictor of SVR in patients with HCV undergoing antiviral treatment, and thus, shorter antiviral treatment for these patients has been suggested.

115 patients with PNALT were enrolled in this study. RVR was observed in 68% of the patients (42% patients with HCV-1, 90% HCV-2 and 64% HCV-3). An end-of-treatment response (EoTR) was observed in 86% of the patients (68% HCV-1, 100% HCV-2 and 91% HCV-3). SVR was maintained in 91 patients (46% HCV-1, 97% HCV-2 and 82% HCV-3). Overall, 92% patients with rapid response did obtain HCV eradication vs only 38% of those without rapid response. HCV-1 patients with baseline HCV RNA <400 x 10^3 IU/mL were more likely to achieve RVR and SVR than those with higher HCV RNA levels. The authors did conclude that patients with genotype 1 and normal ALT who achieve HCV RNA negativity at week 4 may have a higher probability of eradicating their infection.

Because of the concomitant favourable demographic and virological features often found in this particular subset of patients, the duration of therapy in these people might be shortened in the case of RVR. Patients with genotype 2 or 3 have a high chance of achieving SVR, so retesting of HCV RNA during treatment may have no additional practical value in these subjects.

Recently, it has been reported that a 2 log drop in HCV RNA at day 28 was the best predictor of SVR in patients with HCV-1 infection and PNALT treated with PEG-IFN α 2 b plus RBV, and that a failure to reduce viral load by 2 logs correctly identified patients with a low (<15%) probability of achieving a SVR [70].

Finally, the possibility of SVR following extremely short antiviral treatment (5.5 ± 1.5 weeks of treatment with PEG-IFN α 2a plus RBV800 mg/day) has been reported in a selected population of females with HCV-2 chronic infection and PNALT [71].

On the basis of these findings, the Medical Position Statement on the Management of Hepatitis C by the American Gastroenterological Association (AGA) have noted that *"decision analyses in patients with biochemically and histologically mild chronic hepatitis C have led to the conclusion that, even in this population, antiviral therapy is cost-effective. Clinicians may rely in their decision making on individual patient features, including patient motivation and perspective, genotype, relative histologic activity and fibrosis, duration of HCV infection, age, occupation, symptoms, and so on. Recommendation category: I"* [16].

More recently, the American Association for the Study of Liver Disease (AASLD) Practice Guidelines [2] suggest that "While on average, persons with persistently normal ALT values have significantly less liver fibrosis than persons whose ALT levels are abnormal, there are reports of marked fibrosis (5%-30%) and even cirrhosis (1.3%) in persons with normal ALT values. Thus, it is evident that HCV-infected persons with normal ALT values do warrant treatment if the liver biopsy shows significant fibrosis. Moreover, there are multiple studies that report SVR rates with standard-of-care treatment that do not differ from those achieved in persons with abnormal enzymes, and that treatment is equally as safe", thus offering the following recommendations:

a)   Regardless of the serum ALT level, the decision to initiate therapy with PEG-IFN and RBV should be individualized based on the severity of liver disease by liver biopsy, the potential for serious side effects, the likelihood of response, and the presence of comorbid conditions (Class I, Level B).

b)   The treatment regimen for HCV-infected persons with normal aminotransferase levels should be the same as that used for persons with elevated serum aminotransferase levels (Class I, Level B) [2].

In the next future, further studies should address the possibility that PNALT patients might be offered shorter schedules of therapy.

10. MANAGEMENT OF HCV CARRIERS WITH PNALT IN THE CLINICAL PRACTICE

The controversy on the decision whether to treat or not patients with PNALT has been well exemplified by a recent survey performed by the New England Journal of Medicine [72]. The Journal presented a case of a black woman incidentally found to be infected with HCV in Clinical Decisions, an interactive feature designed to assess how readers would manage a clinical problem for which there may be more than one appropriate approach to treatment. The patient was a 25-year-old investment banker who had a positive result on an HCV antibody test when attempting to donate blood for the first time. She was in good health with no other known medical illnesses. She was seronegative for human immunodeficiency virus.

A total of 3216 votes were cast that could be attributed to a continent or region. Of the three treatment options proposed, the most popular — with 1400 votes (44% of the 3216 votes cast) — was the option to perform a liver biopsy and to base further treatment on the findings of the biopsy. The second most popular option, expectant management with periodic assessment of liver function, received 1086 votes (34% of the total), and the option to commence HCV therapy with PEG-IFN and RBV received 708 votes (22% of the total). The 3216 voters were from 115 different countries; the majority of them were from the United States (45%), followed by Italy (5%), the United Kingdom (4%), and Brazil (3%).

The votes and comments to this case reflect the complexities related to the management of HCV infection and the difficulty of balancing commonly encountered treatment-limiting side effects and suboptimal response rates with the potential complications of untreated chronic infection.

Due to the huge number of HCV chronically infected persons with normal ALT levels, priority needs to be defined; it is really impossible to perform liver biopsy in all HCV patients with PNALT, and the cost of treating all these people would be exceedingly high. Thus, the cost-to-benefit ratio should be carefully evaluated, in order to suggest practice guidelines for the everyday management of these subjects [73, 74].

Cost/benefit might be particularly favourable in:

a)   *Young, easy to treat patients (these subjects might have high rate of SVR with short therapy)*

b)   *Middle age patients with "significant" liver disease (at risk of developing end stage liver disease.*

It means that the age issue has a critical role for the decision making [74]. Younger patients have a higher chance to achieve SVR and tolerate therapy better; they have longer life expectancy, are often well motivated, usually have minimal disease and have fewer contraindications. Thus, in this group decision to treat should be based more on expected response and motivation than on the severity of liver disease.

On the contrary, older patients respond less well to therapy, more frequently have significant liver disease and/or co-factors, often have longer infection/disease duration, may experience more side effects and might be less motivated. Thus, in this group decision to treat should be based on the severity of liver disease and on the possibility of sustained response.

How to decide in clinical practice? An Italian Expert Opinion Meeting (endorsed by Italian Association for the Study of the Liver, AISF; Italian Society for the Study of Infectious Diseases, SIMIT; Italian Society for the Study of Sexual Transmitted Diseases, SIMAST) suggested the following recommendations [75]:

a) *Due to the fluctuating pattern of ALT levels in patients with chronic hepatitis C, only more stringent tests will make it possible to distinguish subjects with PNALT from those in transient biochemical remission. The definition of PNALT should be based on at least nine ALT determinations made at intervals of at least 2 months over an 18-month observation period. The optimal ALT threshold should be set at 30 U/L for males and 20 U/L for females (B-II).*

b) *HCV carriers with PNALT may receive antiviral treatment with PEG-IFN plus RBV using the same algorithms and protocols as those recommended for HCV patients with abnormal ALT levels (A-II).*

c) *Decision making should rely on individual characteristics such as genotype, histology, age, potential disease progression, the probability of viral eradication, patient motivation, the desire for pregnancy, comorbidities, co-factors, etc. (A-VI).*

d) *Antiviral treatment might be offered without the need for liver biopsy in patients with a high likelihood of achieving an SVR (e.g. an age of <50 years + easy-to-treat HCV genotype + low viral load), in the absence of any contraindication and co-factors of poor responsiveness (A-VI).*

e) *In patients aged 50-65 years, and in those with a reduced likelihood of achieving an SVR, a liver biopsy may be used to evaluate the need for therapy, with treatment being recommended only for patients with more severe fibrosis (>F2) and a higher possibility of response, depending on the HCV genotype (A-VI).*

f) *Biopsy and therapy are not recommended in therapy elderly (>70 years). These patients should be recommended to adopt lifestyle changes and undergo periodic ALT determinations (D-VI).*

g) *Non-invasive assessments of fibrosis can be used to detect changes over time and consequently indicate the need for biopsy or treatment on an individual patient basis.*

h) *In patients not receiving antiviral treatment, periodic ALT measurements and adequate lifestyles should be recommended. In particular, overweight and the use of alcohol should be strongly discouraged.*

Furthermore, eradication of HCV with PEG-IFN plus RBV is associated with better quality of life and less fatigue in normal ALT patients. These patient benefits, coupled with the high probability of eradicating HCV, should be considered in making decisions about treating this population.

The impact of antiviral treatment with PEG-IFN plus RBV on morbidity and mortality in patients with chronic hepatitis C and PNALT has been evaluated in a recent study from France [76]. Antiviral treatment of HCV-infected populations might reduce 2008-2025 HCV-related morbidity and mortality by 3000 cases of cirrhosis (22%, 2000-5000), 1200 complications (15%, 1000-1700), and 1000 deaths (14%, 900-1300) in the normal ALT population, despite a probability of receiving treatment that is three to five times less in this population. If the HCV patients with normal ALT levels are treated at the same proportions as those with abnormal ALT, morbidity and mortality could be further reduced by 1400 cases of cirrhosis (13%, 1200-2200), 600 complications (9%, 600-1000), and 500 deaths (9%, 500-800). The authors conclude that treatment of PNALT patients would decrease HCV morbidity and mortality, and that these patients should be considered candidates for treatment just as others are.

Thus, regardless of ALT levels, treatment decisions should be individualized based on the severity of liver disease, the potential for serious side effects, the likelihood of treatment response, the presence of comorbid conditions, and the patient's readiness for treatment [2, 17]. In particular, decision making should rely on individual patient features, such as genotype, histology, age of the patient, potential progression of disease, probability of viral eradication, co-morbid illness and co-factors, risk of HCV transmission, patient motivation, desire for pregnancy, quality of life and social or psychological stigma, major concerns over infectivity, etc [2].

In the next future, the use of antiviral agents (HCV polymerase or protease inhibitors) to the current combination therapy will greatly improve SVR rates in patients with CHC and PNALT.

11. CONCLUSION

a) Approximately 30% of patients with chronic HCV infection show persistently normal ALT levels. It is now widely accepted that many of these subjects have some degree of histological liver damage, sometime severe, and the possibility of progression to cirrhosis and liver cancer has been reported.

b) The "classical "definition of persistently normal ALT levels should be made on the basis of at least three normal ALT values 2 months apart over a 6-month period; however, as in clinical practice sudden increases in ALT levels are not uncommon, even at interval longer than 6 months, the optimal observation period should not be shorter than 12-18 months, and ALT determinations should be performed every 2-3 months.

c) The severity of the disease and the progression to more severe liver fibrosis seem to be more frequent in males, in elderly, and in patients showing co-factors for liver damage, such as overweight, liver steatosis, alcohol abuse, co-infection with the Hepatitis B virus (HBV). By contrast, no correlations exist between the severity of liver damage and virological features (HCV genotype, viral load).

d) Given the high rates of sustained virological responses seen with the new combined antiviral therapy (PEG-IFN plus RBV), the risk/benefit ratio became excellent even in patients with benign or slowly progressing disease. Thus, the decision to initiate antiviral treatment should be individualized based on the severity of liver disease by liver biopsy, the potential for serious side effects, the likelihood of response, and the presence of comorbid conditions, rather than on aminotransferase levels.

e) Younger patients have a higher chance to achieve SVR and tolerate therapy better; they have longer life expectancy, are often well motivated, usually have minimal disease and have fewer contraindications. Thus, in this group decision to treat should be based more on expected response and motivation than on the severity of liver disease.

f) Older patients respond less well to therapy, more frequently have significant liver disease and/or co-factors, often have longer infection/disease duration, may experience more side effects and might be less motivated. Thus, in this group decision to treat should be based on the severity of liver disease and on the possibility of sustained response.

REFERENCES

[1]   Strader DB, Wright T, Thomas DL, Seef LB. Diagnosis, management and treatment of hepatitis C. AASLD practice guideline. Hepatology 2004; 39: 1147-71.

[2]   Ghany MG, Strader DB, Thomas DL, Seef LB. Diagnosis, management, and treatment of hepatitis C: an update. Hepatology 2009; 49: 1335-73.

[3]   Puoti C. Hepatitis C with normal aminotransferase levels. Dig Dis 2007; 25: 277-8.

[4]   Puoti C. HCV carriers with persistently normal aminotransferase levels: normal does not always mean healthy. J Hepatol 2003; 38: 529-32.

[5]   Bacon BR. Treatment of patients with Hepatitis C and normal serum aminotransferase levels. Hepatology 2002; 36: S179-84.

[6]   Puoti C, Castellacci R, Montagnese F. Hepatitis C virus carriers with normal aminotransferase levels: healthy people or true patients? Dig Liver Dis 2000; 32: 634-43.

[7]   Martinot-Peignoux M, Boyer N, Cazals-Hatem D, *et al*. Perspective study of anti hepatitis C virus-positive patients with persistently normal serum ALT with or without detectable serum HCV RNA. Hepatology 2001; 34: 1000-5.

[8]   Puoti C, Magrini A, Stati T, *et al*. Clinical, histological and virological features of hepatitis C virus carriers with persistently normal aminotransferase levels. Hepatology 1997; 26: 1393-8.

[9]   Puoti C, Magrini A, Stati T, *et al*. Liver histology in anti-HCV positive subjects with normal ALT levels. Ital J Gastroenterol Hepatol 1997; 29: 383-4.

[10] McLindon JP, Paver MK, Babbs C, Yates AD, *et al*. Hepatitis C-related chronic liver disease among asymptomatic blood donors in the North West of England. J Infect 1995; 30: 253-9.

[11]   Castera L, Foucher J, Bertet J, *et al.* FibroScan and FibroTest to assess liver fibrosis in HCV with normal aminotransferases. Hepatology 2006; 43: 373-4.

[12]   Mathurin P, Moussali J, Cadranel JF, *et al.* Slow progression rate of fibrosis in hepatitis C virus patients with persistently normal alanine aminotransferase activity. Hepatology 1998; 27: 868-72

[13]   Marcellin P, Levy S, Erlinger S. Therapy of hepatitis C: patients with normal aminotransferase levels. Hepatology 1997; 26: 133S-6S.

[14]   Tassopoulos NC. Treatment in patients with normal ALT levels. European Association for the Study of the Liver (EASL) International Consensus Conference on Hepatitis C, Paris, February 26-27, 1999. J Hepatol 1999; 30: 956-61.

[15]   Puoti C, Bellis L, Guarisco R, *et al.* HCV carriers with normal alanine aminotransferase levels: healthy persons or severely ill patients? Eur J Intern Med 2010; 21: 57-61.

[16]   Dienstag JL, McHutchison JG. American Gastroenterological Association [AGA] Medical Position Statement on the Management of Hepatitis C. Gastroenterology 2006; 130: 225-64

[17]   Puoti C, Guido M, Mangia A, *et al.* Committee on HCV carriers with normal alanine aminotransferase levels of the Italian Association for the Study of the Liver. Clinical management of HCV carriers with normal ALT levels. Digest Liver Dis 2003; 35: 362-9.

[18]   Zeuzem S, Alberti A, Rosenberg W, *et al.* Management of patients with chronic hepatitis C virus infection and 'normal' aminotransferase activity. Aliment Pharmacol Ther 2006; 24: 1133-49.

[19]   Puoti C, Bellis L, Martellino F, *et al.* Surveillance of patients with chronic hepatitis C not on antiviral therapy: a practical approach. R J Gastroenterol 2005;14: 141-6

[20]   Zapata R. Clinical approach to the patient with chronic hepatitis C infection and normal aminotransferase. Ann Hepatol 2010; 9: S72-S9.

[21]   Prati D, Taioli E, Zanella A, *et al.* Updated definitions of healthy ranges for serum alanine aminotransferase. Ann Intern Med 2002; 137: 1-10.

[22]   Piton A, Poynard T, Imbert-Bismut F, *et al.* Factors associated with serum alanine aminotransferase activity in healthy subjects: consequences for the definition of normal values, for selection of blood donors, and for patients with chronic hepatitis C. Hepatology 1998; 27: 1213-9.

[23]   Gordon SC, Fang JWS, Silverman A, *et al.* The significance of baseline serum alanine aminotransferase on pretreatment disease characteristics and response to antiviral therapy in chronic hepatitis C. Hepatology 2000; 32: 400-4.

[24]   Puoti C, Guarisco R, Bellis L, Spilabotti L. Diagnosis, management, and treatment of hepatitis C. Hepatology 2009; 50: 322-3.

[25]   Puoti C, Castellacci R, Montagnese F, *et al.* Histological and virological features and follow-up of hepatitis C virus carriers with normal aminotransferase levels: the Italian prospective study of the asymptomatic C carriers (ISACC). J Hepatol 2002; 37: 117-23

[26]   Rumi MG, De Filippi F, Donato MF, *et al.* Progressive hepatic fibrosis in healthy carriers of hepatitis C virus with a aminotransferase breakthrough. J Viral Hepat 2002; 9: 71-4.

[27]   Bellentani S, Tiribelli C, Saccoccio G, *et al.* Prevalence of chronic liver disease in the general population of Northern Italy: The Dyonisos Study. Hepatology 1994; 20: 1442-9

[28]   Stroffolini T, Menchinelli M, Taliani G, *et al.* High prevalence of hepatitis C virus infection in a small central Italian town: lack of evidence of parenteral exposure. Ital J Gastroenterol 1995; 26: 235-8.

[29]   Guadagnino V, Stroffolini T, Rapicetta M, *et al.* Prevalence, risk factors, and genotype distribution of Hepatitis C Virus infection in the general population: a community-based-survey in Southern Italy. Hepatology 1997; 26: 1006-11.

[30]   Puoti C, Pannullo A, Annovazzi G, *et al.* Prevalence of anti Hepatitis C Antibodies among patients hospitalized in a Medical Unit. Eur J Gastroenterol Hepatol 1994; 6: 731-2.

[31]   Alberti A, Morsica G, Chemello L, *et al.* Hepatitis C viraemia and liver disease in symptom-free individuals with anti-HCV. Lancet 1992; 340: 697-8.

[32]   Prieto M, Olaso V, Verdu C, *et al.* Does the healthy hepatitis C virus carrier state really exist? An analysis using Polymerase Chain Reaction. Hepatology 1995; 22: 413-7.

[33]   Shakil AO, Conry-Cantilena C, Alter HJ, *et al.* Volunteer blood donors with antibody to hepatitis C virus: clinical, biochemical, virologic, and histologic features. Ann Intern Med 1995; 123: 330-7.

[34]   Jamal MM, Sony A, Quinn PG, *et al.* Clinical features of Hepatitis C-infected patients with persistently normal alanine aminotransferase levels in the Southwestern United States. Hepatology 1999; 30: 1307-11.

[35]   Serfaty L, Chazouillères O, Pawlotski JM, *et al.* Interferon α therapy in patients with chronic hepatitis C and persistently normal aminotransferase activity. Gastroenterology 1996; 110: 291-5.

[36]   Shiffman ML, Diago M, Tran A, *et al.* Chronic Hepatitis C in patients with persistently normal alanine aminotransferase levels. Clin Gastronterol Hepatol 2006; 6: 645-52.

[37]   Buscarini E, Tanzi E, Zanetti AR, *et al.* High prevalence of antibodies to hepatitis C Virus among family members of patients with anti-HCV-positive chronic liver disease. Scand J Gastroenterol 1993; 28: 343-6.

[38]   Puoti C, Magrini A, Filippi T, Aldegheri L. Do symptomless HCV carriers spread infection to their relatives? Lancet 1995; 346: 843.

[39]   Prati D, Capelli C, Zanella A, *et al.* Influence of different hepatitis C virus genotypes on the course of asymptomatic hepatitis C virus infection. Gastroenterology 1996; 110: 178-83.

[40]   Silini E, Bono F, Cividini A, *et al.* Differential distribution of hepatitis C virus genotypes in patients with and without liver function abnormalities. Hepatology 1995; 21: 285-90.

[41]   Shindo M, Arai K, Sokawa Y, Okuno T. The virological and histological states of anti-hepatitis C virus-positive subjects with normal liver biochemical values. Hepatology 1995; 22: 418-25.

[42]   Nousbaum J-B, Pol S, Nalpas B, *et al.* Hepatitis C virus type 1b (II) infection in France and Italy. Ann Intern Med 1995; 122: 161-8.

[43]   Puoti C, Stati T, Magrini A. Serum HCV RNA titer does not predict the severity of liver damage in HCV carriers with normal aminotransferase levels. Liver 1999; 19: 104-9.

[44]   Pradat P, Alberti A, Poynard T, *et al.* Predictive value of ALT levels for histologic findings in chronic hepatitis C: a European Collaborative Study. Hepatology 2002; 36: 973-7.

[45]   Brambilla S, Bellati G, Asti M, *et al.* Dynamics of hypervariable region 1 in hepatitis C infection and correlation with clinical and virological features of liver disease. Hepatology 1998; 27: 1678-86.

[46]   Hayashi J, Kishihara Y, Yamaji K, *et al.* Hepatitis C viral quasi species and liver damage in patients with chronic hepatitis C virus infection. Hepatology 1997; 25: 697-701.

[47]   Persico M, Persico E, Suozzo R, *et al.* Natural history of hepatitis C virus carriers with persistently normal aminotransferase levels. Gastroenterology 2000; 118:760-4.

[48]   Renou C, Halfon P, Pol S, *et al.* Histological features and HLA class II alleles in HCV chronically infected patients with persistently normal alanine aminotransferase levels. Gut 2002; 51: 585-90.

[49]   Hui C-K, Belaye T, Montegrande K, Wright TL. A comparison in the progression of liver fibrosis in chronic hepatitis C between persistently normal and elevated aminotransferase. J Hepatol 2003; 38: 511-7.

[50]   Puoti C, Bellis L, Galossi A, *et al.* Antiviral treatment of HCV carriers with normal ALT. Mini Rev Med Chem 2008; 8: 150-2.

[51]   Okanoue T, Itoh Y, Minami M, *et al.* Guidelines for the antiviral therapy of hepatitis C virus carriers with normal serum aminotransferase based on platelet counts. Hepatol Res 2008; 38: 27-36.

[52]   Puoti C, Bellis L, Guarisco R. Liver biopsy in Hepatitis C carriers with persistently normal ALT levels. Hepatology 2009; 50: 655-6.

[53]   Ghany MG, Kleiner DE, Alter H, *et al.* Progression of fibrosis in chronic hepatitis C. Gastroenterology 2003; 124: 97-104.

[54]   Lawson A, for the Trent Hepatitis C Study Group. Hepatitis C virus-infected patients with a persistently normal alanine aminotransferase: do they exist and is this really a group with mild disease? J Viral Hepat. 2010; 17: 51-8

[55]   Okanoue T, Makiyama A, Nakayama M, *et al.* A follow-up study to determine the value of liver biopsy and need for antiviral therapy for hepatitis C virus carriers with persistently normal serum aminotransferase. J Hepatol 2005; 43: 599-605.

[56]   Cividini A, Rebucci C, Silini E, Mondelli MU. Is the natural history of HCV carriers with normal aminotransferase levels really benign? Gastroenterology 2001; 121:1526-7.

[57]   Persico M, Palmentieri B, Coppola L, *et al.* Occurrence of HCC in asymptomatic HCV-related chronic hepatitis. Digest Dis Sci 2002; 47: 2407-10.

[58]   Puoti C, Bellis L, Martellino F, *et al.* Occurrence of hepatocellular carcinoma in an apparently 'healthy' HCV patient. Eur J Gastroenterol Hepatol 2005; 17: 1263-4.

[59]   Kobayashi M, Suzuki F, Akuta N, *et al.* Development of hepatocellular carcinoma in elderly patients with chronic hepatitis C with or without elevated aspartate and alanine aminotransferase levels. J Hepatol. 2009; 50: 729-35.

[60]   Van Thiel DH, Caraceni P, Molloy PJ, *et al.* Chronic hepatitis C in patients with normal or near normal alanine aminotransferase levels: the role of interferon α 2b therapy. J Hepatol 1995; 23: 503-8.

[61] Sangiovanni A, Morales R, Spinzi GC, *et al.* Interferon α treatment of HCV RNA carriers with persistently normal aminotransferase levels: a pilot randomized controlled study. Hepatology 1998; 27: 853-6.

[62] Rossini A, Ravaggi A, Biasi L, *et al.* Virological response to interferon treatment in hepatitis C virus carriers with normal aminotransferase levels and chronic hepatitis. Hepatology 1997; 26: 1012-7.

[63] Lee SS, Sherman M. Pilot study of interferon-α and ribavirin treatment in patients with chronic hepatitis C and normal aminotransferase values. J Viral Hepat 2001; 8: 202-5.

[64] Hui CK, Monto A, Belaye T, *et al.* Outcomes of interferon α and ribavirin treatment for chronic hepatitis C in patients with normal serum aminoaminotransferases. Gut 2003; 52: 1644-8.

[65] Jacobson IM, Ahmed F, Russo MW, *et al.* Interferon α-2b and ribavirin for patients with chronic hepatitis C and normal ALT. Am J Gastroenterol 2004; 99: 1700-5.

[66] Zeuzem S, Diago M, Gane E, *et al.* Peginterferon α-2a [40KD] and ribavirin in patients with chronic hepatitis C and normal aminotransferase levels. Gastroenterology 2004; 127:1724-32.

[67] Snoeck E, Hadziyannis SJ, Puoti C, *et al.* Predicting efficacy and safety outcomes inpatients with hepatitis C virus genotype 1 and persistently 'normal' alanine aminotransferase levels treated with Peginterferon α-2a (40KD) plus ribavirin. Liver Int 2008; 28: 61-71.

[68] Puoti C, Pellicelli A, Romano M, *et al.* Treatment of hepatitis C virus carriers with persistently normal alanine aminotransferase levels with Peginterferon alfa-2a and ribavirin: a multicentric study. Liver Int 2009; 29: 1479-84.

[69] Puoti C, Barbarini G, Picardi A, *et al.*, on behalf of the Club Epatologico Ospedaliero (Hospital Liver Club, CLEO). Rapid virological response as a predictor of sustained response in HCV-infected patients with persistently normal alanine aminotransferase levels: A multicenter study. J Viral Hepat. 2010 (in press, doi:10.1111/j.1365-2893.2010.01319.x).

[70] Deltenre P, Canva V, El Nady M, *et al.* A 2-log drop in viral load at 1 month is the best predictor of sustained response in HCV patients with normal ALT: a kinetic prospective study. J Viral Hepat. 2009; 16: 500-5.

[71] Puoti C, Guarisco R, Spilabotti L, Bellis L. Sustained virological response following extremely short antiviral treatment in selected HCV carriers with persistently normal ALT. Digest Liver Dis 2010; 42: 745 (letter).

[72] Afdhal NH, Lok AS, Di Bisceglie AM. Management of incidental hepatitis C virus infection. N Engl J Med 2009; 360: 1902-6.

[73] Puoti C. Antiviral treatment of HCV-related chronic hepatitis: is the cup half empty, or half full? J Gastrointest Liver Dis 2007;16 :171-2.

[74] Alberti A. Towards a more individualised management of HCV patients with initially or persistently normal alanine aminotransferase levels. J Hepatol 2005; 42: 266-74.

[75] Practice guidelines for the treatment of hepatitis C: Recommendations from an AISF/SIMIT/SIMAST Expert Opinion Meeting. Digest Liver Dis 2010; 42: 81-91.

[76] Deuffic-Burban S, Babany G, Lonjon-Domanec I, *et al.* Impact of Pegylated interferon and ribavirin on morbidity and mortality in patients with chronic hepatitis C and normal aminotransferases in France. Hepatology 2009; 50:1351-9.

CHAPTER 5

Innate Immune Response and Sex Hormones

Yoshiki Katakura, Tsutoshi Asaki, Yosho Fukita and Ichiro Shimizu*

Department of Gastroenterology, Seirei Yokohama Hospital, 215 Iwai-cho, Hodogaya-ku, Kanagawa 240-8521, Japan

Abstract: Females are more resistant to certain infections, and suffer a higher incidence of autoimmune diseases. Immune disease expression is also affected by the reproductive status of the female. Indeed, the decline in ovarian function with menopause is associated with spontaneous increase in pro-inflammatory cytokines, tumor necrosis factor-α (TNF-α), interleukin-1 and interleukin-6. In general, estradiol seems to have anti-inflammatory effects on neutrophils, while progesterone seems to have pro-inflammatory effects on these cells. In males an increase in blood monocyte number is demonstrated as compared to females during menopause in the follicular phase. Increased potency to lyse other cells is found in postmenopausal females and in males as compared to females with a regular menstrual cycle. This is in line with the fact that natural killer (NK) cell activity is also decreased in postmenopausal females using hormone replacement therapy. *In vitro* estrogens appear to suppress NK cell activity. Estrogens appear to increase the numbers and function of regulatory T lymphocytes, which inhibit the adaptive immune response. In contrast, progesterone may counteract the estrogen effects. Sex differences in immune responses therefore account for, at least in part, the sex differences in incidence and progression of liver disease.

Keywords: TNF-α, interleukin-1, interleukin-6, estradiol, progesterone, testosterone, menopause, hormone replacement therapy, cytotoxic T cell, NK cell, regulatory T cell, immune system.

1. INTRODUCTION

Females are more resistant to certain infections, and suffer a higher incidence of autoimmune diseases. Immune disease expression is also affected by the reproductive status of the female. There are two arms of the immune system, the innate (natural or non-specific) immune system and the adaptive (specific or acquired) immune system. The adaptive immune system is activated by the innate immune response, and specifically responded by pathogen and antigen. One of the key features of the innate immune response is tissue inflammation by inflammatory. The decline in ovarian function with menopause is associated with spontaneous increase in pro-inflammatory cytokines, such as tumor necrosis factor-α (TNF-α), interleukin-1 (IL-1) and interleukin-6 (IL-6) [1]. The effector cells of the innate immune response are monocytes, macrophages, neutrophils, and natural killer (NK) cells. In general, estradiol seems to have anti-inflammatory effects on such cells, while another sex steroid hormone, progesterone seems to have pro-inflammatory effects on the cells [2,3]. Progesterone has some structural and functional similarities to male sex hormone testosterone [2].

Moreover, the cellular components of the adaptive immune response are T lymphocytes and B lymphocytes. Cytotoxic T lymphocyte (Tc cell) function may play a role in the differences in progression of liver disease between males and females. Regulatory T cells (Treg cells) may inhibit the adaptive immune response during the progression phase and thereby limit tissue destruction and progression of the liver disease. The aim of this chapter is to describe the effects of sex hormones, estrogens, progesterone and testosterone, on immune responses.

2. BIOSYNTHESIS OF ESTROGENS, PROGESTERONE AND ANDROGENS

The ovarian steroids are synthesized from cholesterol *via* pregnenolone by essentially the same pathways as exist in other steroid-producing organs such as the testis, adrenal cortex, and placenta.

*Address correspondence to Ichiro Shimizu:** Department of Gastroenterology, Seirei Yokohama Hospital, 215 Iwai-cho, Hodogaya-ku, Yokohama, Kanagawa 240-8521, Japan; Tel: +81-45-715-3111; Fax: +81-45-715-3387; E-mail: ichiro.shimizu@showaclinic.jp

The principal estrogen secreted by the ovary and the most potent naturally occurring estrogen is estradiol. Estrone is also secreted by the ovary, but the principal source of estrone is from extraglandular conversion of androstenedione in peripheral tissues such as adipose tissue. Estriol, the most abundant estrogen in urine, arises from the 16-hydroxylation of estrone and estradiol in urine. The liver is the principal site of the interconversion of estradiol and estrone. Progesterone is the primary hormone secreted by the corpus luteum and is responsible for progestational effects. The liver is largely responsible for the inactivation of estrogens and progesterone. Hormonal fluctuations in the menstrual cycle include increasing estradiol, but low progesterone blood concentrations in the follicular phase, and high blood concentrations of estradiol and progesterone in the luteal phase. During the luteal phase, however, the blood concentration of progesterone rises up to a maximum of about 10^{-7} mol/L, which is ten to a hundred times higher than that of estradiol [4].

The ovary synthesizes a variety of 19-carbon steroids, including dehydroepiandrosterone, androstenedione, testosterone, and dihydrotestosterone. The major ovarian 19-carbon steroid is androstenedione, of which is secreted into blood and the remainder of which is converted to estrogens or to testosterone. In peripheral tissues, the most being adipose tissue, androstenedione can be converted to testosterone and to estrogens, and then testosterone also can be converted to dihydrotestosterone. Only testosterone and dihydrotestosterone are true androgens that interact with the androgen receptor and induce virilizing signs in females. Testosterone has some structural and functional similarities to progesterone [2] (Fig. **1**).

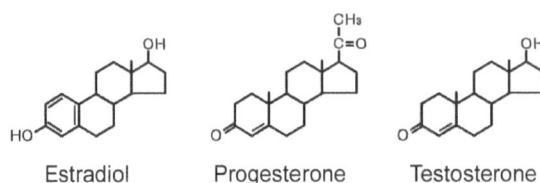

Estradiol   Progesterone   Testosterone

Fig. 1. The structural formulas of natural estradiol, progesterone, and testosterone. Progesterone has some structural similarities to testosterone rather than to estradiol.

3. INNATE IMMUNE RESPONSE AND ADAPTIVE IMMUNE SYSTEM

Both innate and adaptive immunity (Table **1**) depend on the ability of the immune system to distinguish between "self" and "non-self" molecules. In immunology, "self" molecules are those components of an organism body that can be distinguished from foreign substances by the immune system. In contrast, "non-self" molecules are those recognized as foreign molecules. One class of non-self molecules is called antigens and is defined as substances that bind to specific immune receptors and elicit an immune response.

Table 1. Comparison between innate immune system and adaptive immune system

Innate Immune System	Adaptive Immune System
Response is non-specific The first line of defence against infections	Pathogen and antigen specific response Activation by the innate immune response
Exposure leads to immediate maximal response	Lag time between exposure and maximal response
Found in nearly all plants and animals	Found only in jawed vertebrates
Cell-mediated and humoral components	Cell-mediated and humoral components

The innate immune response is the first line of defence against infections. It recognizes structures specific for microbes. The effector cells of the innate immune response are monocytes, macrophages, granulocytes (neutrophils, eosinophils and basophils), dendritic cells and NK cells. These cells attack microbes which have entered the circulation (Table **2**). They do so by phagocytosing the microbe (the effector cells are neutrophils, monocytes and macrophages), by cytolysis of infected cells (NK cells) or by producing cytokines, including pro-inflammatory cytokines and chemokines, to enhance innate and adaptive immune responses (the cells above). One of the key features of the innate immune response is tissue inflammation by inflammatory and phagocytic cells, such as neutrophils, monocytes and macrophages. These cells respond to inflammatory and oxidative stimuli by producing reactive oxygen species (ROS), such as superoxide and hydrogen peroxide. ROS may contribute to inflammatory and phagocytic cell-mediated killing of microbes. Dendritic cells are the most important antigen presenting cell. They take up foreign antigens such as viruses or pathogens, process the antigens and present antigen peptides in the context of major histocompatibility complex (MHC) class II molecules on their surface, and exhibit them to the adaptive immune system, mainly helper T lymphocytes. There are two classes of MHC molecules. An extremely heterogeneous system of molecules found on all cells (MHC class I) or only on B lymphocytes, macrophages and dendritic cells (MHC class II). Their role is to present small antigenic peptides to the T cell receptor (TCR), and the class of MHC and the type of T cell determine the characteristics of the resulting immune response.

Table 2. Definitions of terms and abbreviation on the innate immune system

Innate immune system	Non-specific defence responses by phagocytosing the microbe (the effector cells are neutrophils, monocytes and macrophages), by cytolysis of infected cells (NK cells) or by producing cytokines including pro-inflammatory cytokines and chemokines to enhance innate and adaptive immune responses (the cells above and dendritic cells)
Dendritic cell	Antigen presenting cell, taking up foreign antigens, processing the antigens and presenting antigen peptides in the context of major histocompatibility complex (MHC) II molecules on its surface, and exhibiting them to the specific immune system, mainly helper T lymphocytes
Monocyte	The largest nucleated cell of the blood, developing into a macrophage when it migrates into the tissues
Macrophage	Principal resident phagocyte of the tissues and serous cavities such as the peritoneum; Kupffer cell is the specialized macrophage located in the liver
NK (natural killer) cell	Lymphocyte-like cell capable of killing some targets, notably virus-infected cells and tumor cells, but without the T cell receptor (TCR), by releasing called perforin
Pro-inflammatory cytokine	Cytokine produced predominantly by activated immune cells and involved in the amplification of inflammatory reactions; tumor necrosis factor-α (TNF-α), interleukin-1 (IL-1), interleukin-6 (IL-6)
Chemokine	Cytokine playing a key role in chemotaxis (attracting neutrophils, lymphocytes, monocytes and macrophages to inflammatory sites); monocyte chemoattractant protein-1 (MCP-1), interleukin-8 (IL-8)

 T lymphocytes express the TCR. Two forms of TCRs are now recognized: the $\alpha\beta$ TCR, which is responsible for MHC restricted antigen recognition, and the $\gamma\delta$ TCR, which is not MHC restricted. Within the T lymphocyte population expressing the $\alpha\beta$ TCR, Tc cells (CD8$^+$ cells) can directly kill foreign and infected cells. CD is a classification of the molecules found on the surface of T and B cells, and is used to classify T and B cell subpopulations. Helper T lymphocytes (Th cells) (CD4$^+$ cells) provide help to other immune cells by producing cytokines. The Th cells produce so called Th1 cytokines, such as interferon-γ (IFN-γ) and interleukin-2 (IL-2), which generally promote cellular immune responses. They also produce Th2 cytokines such as interleukin-4 (IL-4), interleukin-5 (IL-5) and interleukin-10 (IL-10) to provide optimal help for humoral immune response. Th cells that can produce Th1 cytokines and Th2 cytokines are called Th0 cells to be precursors for Th1 and Th2 cells. Recently, 2 new populations of Th cells have been identified, namely Th17 cells and regulatory Th cells. Th17 cells appear to play a crucial role in autoimmunity and allergen-specific immune responses [5].

Treg cells, formerly known as suppressor T cells, are now thought to be a central mechanism of immune regulation [6]. Treg cells are divided into a natural CD4$^+$CD25$^+$ Treg cell population and diverse populations of induced (or adaptive) Treg cells. Natural Treg cells develop in the thymus under strong TCR engagement with self peptides and play an important role in the maintenance of self-tolerance and immune homeostasis. In contrast to natural Treg cells, induced Treg cells develop from non-regulatory Th cells in the periphery and not in the thymus [7]. Based on the phenotype and cytokine profile, Treg cells are currently identified as CD4$^+$CD25$^+$FoxP3$^+$ Tregs, IL-10-producing CD4$^+$ Treg type 1 (Tr1), TGF-β-

producing CD4$^+$ Th3, CD4$^+$CD25$^+$ Tregs converted from activated CD4$^+$CD25$^-$ T cells and IL-10- or transforming growth factor-β (TGF-β)-producing CD8$^+$ T cells, and a minor subset of CD4$^+$CD25$^-$ cells [8]. TGF-β is a potent fibrogenic cytokine, regulating the production, degradation and accumulation of the extracellular matrix in hepatic fibrosis. In addition, TGF-β has also the additional properties of inhibiting cellular immunity and regulating production of IgA and IgE by B cells. The major function of natural and induced Treg cells is the suppression of immune responses to self or foreign antigens.

4. INNATE IMMUNE RESPONSE AND SEX HORMONES

In inflammatory and oxidative liver injury, the accumulation of neutrophils, lymphocytes, monocytes and macrophages including Kupffer cells to sites of inflammation and injury is thought to be mediated by chemokines, such as monocyte chemoattractant protein-1 (MCP-1) and interleukin-8 (IL-8). Chemokines are a subset of cytokines, which attract and activate immune cells. Monocytes develop into macrophages when they migrate into the tissues. Kupffer cells are the specialized macrophages located in the liver. The inflammatory cells such as neutrophils, monocytes and macrophages are in turn able to release pro-inflammatory cytokines, including TNF-α, IL-1 and IL-6, as well as ROS, leading to cell death and persistent liver injury (Fig. **2**). Liver cell (hepatocyte) destruction derives from such actions as lipid peroxidation and DNA injury by ROS, apoptosis by TNF-α, and phagocytosis by inflammatory cells.

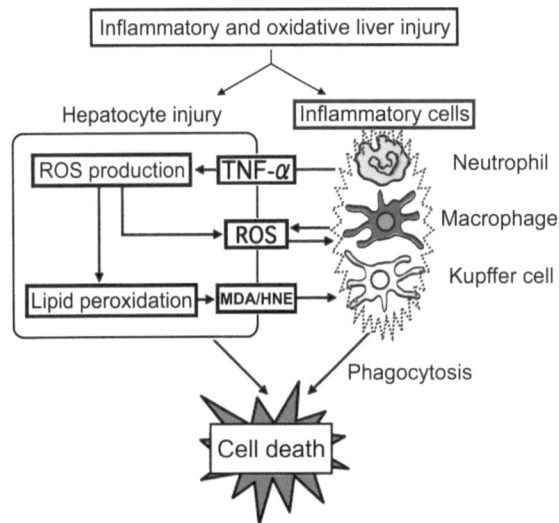

Fig. 2. In inflammatory and oxidative liver injury, liver cell (hepatocyte) destruction derives from such actions as lipid peroxidation and DNA injury by reactive oxygen species (ROS), apoptosis by TNF-α, and phagocytosis by inflammatory cells (neutrophils, macrophages and Kupffer cells). Destructed hepatocytes release ROS and end products of lipid peroxidation, malondialdehyde (MDA) and 4-hydroxynonenal (HNE), which also activate inflammatory cells. Activated inflammatory cells produce TNF-α and ROS.

Neutrophils are the first cells recruited from the bloodstream to sites of infection. The function of neutrophils is mainly phagocytosis. Neutrophils respond to chemotactic stimuli and produce factors, such as ROS, in order to kill the phagocytosed cells. It is reported that estrogens decreased chemotactic activity of neutrophils, while progesterone enhanced this activity [9]. Several studies showed inhibitory effects of estrogens on monocyte MCP-1 production and the MCP-1-induced migration of monocytes [10-12]. In general, estradiol seems to have anti-inflammatory effects on neutrophils, while progesterone seems to have pro-inflammatory effects on these cells.

NK cells are capable of killing virus-infected cells or tumour cells in the absence of prior immunization and without MHC restriction. They lyse target cells by direct contact with them in the absence of antibody or by antibody dependent cellular cytotoxicity (ADCC). Increased potency to lyse other cells is found in postmenopausal females and in males as compared to females with a regular menstrual cycle [13,14]. This is in line with the fact that NK cell activity is also decreased in postmenopausal females using hormone replacement therapy (HRT) [15]. For HRT, estrogen is combined with progestin for women with a uterus to prevent endometrial hyperplasia and endometrial cancer. *In vitro* estrogen appears to suppresse NK cell activity [14,15].

Dendritic cells are specialist antigen presenting cells, which are derived from monocytes and immature dendritic cells reside in the tissues. They serve as a link between innate and adaptive immune responses and are essential for activation and regulation of immune responses against infections. Studies on the different subpopulations of dendritic cells have shown that progesterone inhibits IFN-γ production by plasmacoid dendritic cells. These plasmacoid dendritic cells are circulating and tissue-based dendritic cells that produce large amounts of IFN-γ after encountering viruses. Since IFN-γ induces an antiviral state and primes antiviral response in the adaptive immune response, *via* this mechanisms, progesterone seems to inhibit antiviral responses [16]. In contrast, estradiol induces the production of IFN-γ in lymphocytes [17].

The effects of sex and the reproductive condition upon monocyte cytokine production are obvious. The most important and consistent effects are as follows. Stimulated TNF-α and IL-1 production is increased in males as compared to females, and also increased in the luteal phase as compared to the follicular phase of the ovarian cycle [18]. Hormonal fluctuations in the menstrual cycle include increasing estradiol, but low progesterone blood concentrations in the follicular phase, and high blood concentrations of estradiol and progesterone in the luteal phase. During the luteal phase, however, the blood concentration of progesterone rises up to a maximum, which is ten to a hundred times higher than that of estradiol [4].

There is large body of evidence indicating that the decline in ovarian function with menopause is associated with spontaneous increases in pro-inflammatory cytokines TNF-α, IL-1 and IL-6 [1]. During menopause and in males an increase in blood monocyte number is demonstrated as compared to females in the follicular phase [19]. Moreover, during menopause the monocyte counts decline following estrogen replacement therapy [20]. A very important function of monocytes is to direct immune responses by the production of cytokines including TNF-α, IL-1 and IL-6. Endotoxin-stimulated monocytes in males produce more TNF-α as compared to females [21]. Endotoxins, bacterial lipopolysaccharides in gastrointestinal tract, are detoxified in the reticuloendothelial system, particularly in monocytes-macrophages and Kupffer cells. These cells stimulated by endotoxin induce pro-inflammatory cytokines. Whether the sex difference of TNF-α response to endotoxin is due to direct effects of high levels of testosterone in males remains uncertain since *in vitro* studies showed no effect of testosterone upon monocyte TNF-α production [22]. Higher blood levels of TNF-α and IL-1 are reported during the luteal phase as compared with the follicular phase, while endotoxin-stimulated monocytes from the luteal phase produce more TNF-α and IL-1 as compared with the follicular phase [23,24]. Estrogens can inhibit IL-6 production by Kupffer cells in mice [25]. Increased blood IL-6 levels after menopause are also decreased by HRT [26,27]. Further evaluation indicates that the decrease in blood IL-6 levels is due to the estrogenic component in HRT [26,27], while one study showes that the prostagens in the HRT up-regulate stimulated IL-6 production [28].

As far as the *in vitro* studies with female sex hormones on the pro-inflammatory cytokine production by monocytes are concerned, however, conflicting data have been published [29], varying from some [30-32] to no [21,33] effect of estradiol or progesterone on the cytokine production. Estradiol, at physiological concentrations, has been shown to inhibit the spontaneous secretion of these pro-inflammatory cytokines in whole blood cultures [33] or peripheral blood mononuclear cells (PBMCs) [34]. The spontaneous production of TNF-α and IL-1 by PBMCs is higher in patients with chronic hepatitis C than in healthy subjects [35]. Endotoxin-stimulated TNF-α production by PBMCs is also higher in hepatitis B surface antigen (HBsAg) carriers with elevated levels of alanine aminotransferase (ALT) than in HBsAg carriers with normal ALT levels [36]. Moreover, TNF-α production by hepatocytes from patients with chronic hepatitis B virus (HBV) infection is reported to be transcriptionally up-regulated by hepatitis B x (HBx) protein [37,38]. Treatment with estradiol transdermally in postmenopausal females decreases spontaneous IL-6 production by PBMCs after 12 months of the therapy [34]. Recent studies also show inhibitory effects of estradiol on the unstimulated and hydrogen peroxide-stimulated production of TNF-α, IL-1, IL-8, and MCP-1 in PBMCs from patients with chronic hepatitis C and in murine peritoneal macrophages, whereas progesterone counteract the estradiol effects by enhancing the accumulation of inflammatory cells and their cytokine production [3,39] (Fig. **3**).

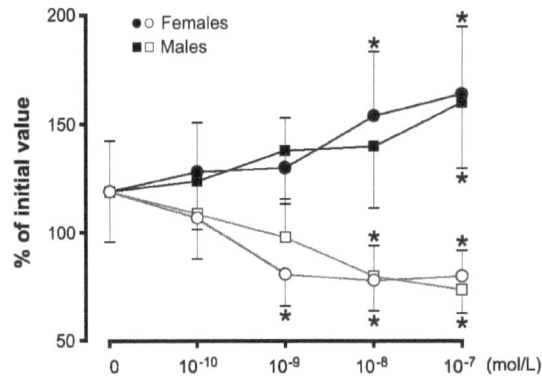

Fig. 3. Estradiol (open) inhibits and progesterone (solid) stimulates spontaneous production of TNF-α by unstimulated peripheral blood mononuclear cells (PBMCs) from age-matched older male (square) and postmenopausal female (circle) patients with chronic hepatitis C [3]. The unstimulated PBMCs were cultured with and without estradiol (10^{-10}-10^{-7} mol/L) or progesterone (10^{-10}-10^{-7} mol/L). The results are expressed as the percentages of each initial value for the cytokine production in the absence of the female sex hormones. The values are the mean ± SD ($n = 18$). $^{*}P < 0.05$ in comparison with the cultures in the absence of the female sex hormones.

In general, the data suggest an inhibition of the innate immune response in females as compared to males. Although a suppression of innate immune responses may inhibit the clearance of the virus in the acute liver infection, decreased production of pro-inflammatory cytokines may be beneficial in the progression of the liver disease. Judging from these findings and the previous data showing that the action for ROS production processes is completely opposite to estradiol (anti-oxidant) with progesterone (pro-oxidant), estradiol may exert a hepatoprotective action against inflammation and oxidative stress in the course of persistent liver injury by preventing the accumulation of neutrophils, monocytes and macrophages and by inhibiting the production of pro-inflammatory cytokines and ROS, whereas progesterone may counteract the favorable estradiol effects (Fig. **4**). Progesterone also resembles testosterone in the part of the structure and function. Therefore, the sex hormones estrogens, progesterone and testosterone may affect innate immune responses by modulating inflammatory cell numbers and function as well as ROS production.

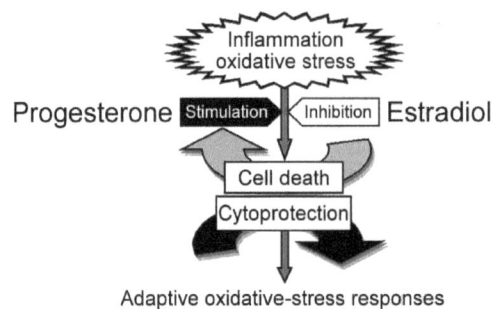

Fig. 4. Adaptive oxidative-stress responses to inflammatory and oxidative stimuli by estradiol and progesterone. For neutrophils, monocytes and macrophages, estradiol exerts anti-inflammatory and antioxidative effects, while progesterone exerts pro-inflammatory and pro-oxidative effects [3,18,39]. The decrease in immune responses by estradiol limits tissue destruction during the inflammatory and oxidative liver injury and thus relatively protects females against the progression of liver disease.

5. ADAPTIVE IMMUNE RESPONSE AND SEX HORMONES

In the peripheral blood about 30% of the white blood cells are lymphocytes. Of these lymphocytes, about 85-90% are T lymphocytes and about 95% of the T lymphocytes express the αβ TCR, of which about 60% are Th lymphocytes, and about 40% are Tc and Treg lymphocytes. Total lymphocyte count in males is similar to females [19], while the percentage of T cells within the total lymphocyte population in males is lower as compared to females [19]. The decreased T-cell counts in males as compared to females may be due to the increased testosterone concentrations, since testosterone may increase apoptosis in T cells [40].

Many studies both *in vitro* and *in vivo* have shown that estrogens suppress cell-mediated immune response [41]. Estrogens inhibit proliferation of T cells (or T lymphocyte cell lines) after stimulation with mitogenic substances [42]. Estrogens decrease TNF-α-induced cytotoxicity in peripheral T cells [43], and they enhance secretion of IL-10 in T cells isolated from females [44]. IL-10 is an inhibitory cytokine serving to limit cell-mediated responses. The inhibitory effect of sex hormones on Tc cell function may play a role in the differences in progression of liver disease between males and females, since, as suggested for neutrophils, monocytes and macrophages, decreased Tc cell cytotoxicity in females as compared to males could limit tissue destruction following acute infection and thereby progression of liver disease. Although there is little information about the direct effects of progesterone on the Tc cell function, progesterone may act in opposition to the favorable effects of estrogens [2,3].

Moreover, females have a higher number of Th cells than males [45]. The main function of Th cells is cytokine production. Estrogens are also reported to enhance humoral immune responses (Th2 cells) [46]. Such effects of estrogens on humoral and cell-mediated immune responses may be modulated by their effects on Th1 and Th2 cytokine production.

B lymphocytes represent 5-15% of circulating lymphocytes. The main function of B cells is the production of antibodies. B cells have two subsets. The first set is the conventional B cell subset (B2 cells), which present internalised antigens to T cells through which they get activated and develop into antibody-producing blood cells (plasma cells) [47]. The second subset is the B1 cell subset, which produce antibodies in a T cell independent manner and are suggested to be responsible for autoantibody production [48]. B1 subsets appear to remaine stable after menopause, while the B2 subset appear to decrease after menopause and to increase after HRT [49]. Studies in animals have shown that estrogens increase bone marrow progenitor B cells in mice by protecting the progenitor cells from apoptosis, and increase survival in splenic B cells [50]. Females, particularly before menopause, can produce antibodies against hepatitis B e antigen (HBeAg) and HBsAg at a higher frequency than males with chronic HBV infection. In addition to the inhibitory effect of estrogens on the cell-mediated immune response, estrogens also enhance B cell development, while androgens appear to inhibit humoral immunity [51]. These may be involved in the higher incidence of autoimmune diseases in females. Indeed, estrogens increased and testosterone decreased autoantibody production of PBMC in patients with systemic lupus erythematosus (SLE) [52], which is one of common autoimmune diseases predominat in females.

The number of CD4$^+$CD25$^+$ Treg cells increase during the late follicular phase, concomitantly with high estradiol concentrations, compared to early follicular phase or luteal phase, while during the luteal phase with high progesterone concentrations there are no changes in numbers of CD4$^+$CD25$^+$ Treg cells between these phases of the ovarian cycle [53,54]. This suggests that high concentrations of estradiol is involved in the increase in numbers of Treg cells. Therefore, estrogens induce the suppressive function of Treg cells for immune responses to self or foreign antigens [53]. It has been shown in mice that estrogens increase expression of Foxp3 present in Treg cells together with Treg cell function [55]. Foxp3 is a transcription factor that controls the development and function of Treg cells [55]. Since Treg cells may inhibit the adaptive immune response during the progression phase and thereby limit tissue destruction and progression of the liver disease, estrogens may also suppress the disease progression *via* affecting adaptive immune responses in the liver. On the other hand, progesterone may counteract the estrogen effects.

6. CONCLUSION

Estrogens may play a favorable role in the course of persistent liver injury, at least, by preventing the accumulation of monocytes and macrophages and by also inhibiting the pro-inflammatory cytokine production, whereas progesterone may act in opposition to these positive estrogen effects by enhancing the accumulation of inflammatory cells and their cytokine production. Moreover, estrogens appear to increase the numbers and function of Treg cells, which inhibit the adaptive immune response. Studies on the effects of sex hormones on Treg cells are limited at the moment, especially the effects on Treg cell subsets and function. Further studies are needed to substantiate this hypothesis [18]. Anyway, sex differences in immune responses therefore account for, at least in part, the sex differences in incidence and progression of liver disease.

REFERENCES

[1] Pfeilschifter J, Koditz R, Pfohl M, Schatz H. Changes in Proinflammatory Cytokine Activity after Menopause. Endocr Rev 2002;23:90-119.

[2] Cheng X, Shimizu I, Yuan Y, *et al.* Effects of estradiol and progesterone on tumor necrosis factor alpha-induced apoptosis in human hepatoma HuH-7 cells. Life Sci 2006;79:1988-94.

[3] Yuan Y, Shimizu I, Shen M, *et al.* Effects of estradiol and progesterone on the proinflammatory cytokine production by mononuclear cells from patients with chronic hepatitis C. World J Gastroenterol 2008;14:2200-7.

[4] Clayton RN, Royston JP, Chapman J, *et al.* Is changing hypothalamic activity important for control of ovulation? Br Med J (Clin Res Ed) 1987;295:7-12.

[5] Harrington LE, Mangan PR, Weaver CT. Expanding the effector CD4 T-cell repertoire: the Th17 lineage. Curr Opin Immunol 2006;18:349-56.

[6] Bluestone JA, Abbas AK. Natural versus adaptive regulatory T cells. Nat Rev Immunol 2003;3:253-7.

[7] Billerbeck E, Bottler T, Thimme R. Regulatory T cells in viral hepatitis. World J Gastroenterol 2007;13:4858-64.

[8] Dolganiuc A, Szabo G. T cells with regulatory activity in hepatitis C virus infection: what we know and what we don't. J Leukoc Biol 2008;84:614-22.

[9] Miyagi M, Aoyama H, Morishita M, Iwamoto Y. Effects of sex hormones on chemotaxis of human peripheral polymorphonuclear leukocytes and monocytes. J Periodontol 1992;63:28-32.

[10] Okada M, Suzuki A, Mizuno K, *et al.* Effects of 17 beta-estradiol and progesterone on migration of human monocytic THP-1 cells stimulated by minimally oxidized low-density lipoprotein *in vitro.* Cardiovasc Res 1997;34:529-35.

[11] Janis K, Hoeltke J, Nazareth M, *et al.* Estrogen decreases expression of chemokine receptors, and suppresses chemokine bioactivity in murine monocytes. Am J Reprod Immunol 2004;51:22-31.

[12] Yada-Hashimoto N, Nishio Y, Ohmichi M, *et al.* Estrogen and raloxifene inhibit the monocytic chemoattractant protein-1-induced migration of human monocytic cells *via* nongenomic estrogen receptor alpha. Menopause 2006;13:935-41.

[13] Houglum K, Brenner DA, Chojkier M. D-alpha-tocopherol inhibits collagen alpha 1(I) gene expression in cultured human fibroblasts. Modulation of constitutive collagen gene expression by lipid peroxidation. J Clin Invest 1991;87:2230-5.

[14] Yovel G, Shakhar K, Ben-Eliyahu S. The effects of sex, menstrual cycle, and oral contraceptives on the number and activity of natural killer cells. Gynecol Oncol 2001;81:254-62.

[15] Stopinska-Gluszak U, Waligora J, Grzela T, *et al.* Effect of estrogen/progesterone hormone replacement therapy on natural killer cell cytotoxicity and immunoregulatory cytokine release by peripheral blood mononuclear cells of postmenopausal women. J Reprod Immunol 2006;69:65-75.

[16] Hughes GC, Thomas S, Li C, *et al.* Cutting edge: progesterone regulates IFN-alpha production by plasmacytoid dendritic cells. J Immunol 2008;180:2029-33.

[17] Fox HS, Bond BL, Parslow TG. Estrogen regulates the IFN-gamma promoter. J Immunol 1991;146:4362-7.

[18] Faas MM, Bouman A, de Vos P. The immune response in humans is affected by the sex hormones estrogens, progesterone and testosterone. In: Shimizu I, ed. Female Hepatology: Impact of female sex against progression of liver disease, Kerala, India: Research Signpost, 2009.

[19] Bouman A, Schipper M, Heineman MJ, Faas MM. Gender difference in the non-specific and specific immune response in humans. Am J Reprod Immunol 2004;52:19-26.

[20] Ben-Hur H, Mor G, Insler V, *et al.* Menopause is associated with a significant increase in blood monocyte number and a relative decrease in the expression of estrogen receptors in human peripheral monocytes. Am J Reprod Immunol 1995;34:363-9.

[21] Bouman A, Schipper M, Heineman MJ, Faas M. 17beta-estradiol and progesterone do not influence the production of cytokines from lipopolysaccharide-stimulated monocytes in humans. Fertil Steril 2004;82 Suppl 3:1212-9.

[22] Posma E, Moes H, Heineman MJ, Faas MM. The effect of testosterone on cytokine production in the specific and non-specific immune response. Am J Reprod Immunol 2004;52:237-43.

[23] Bouman A, Moes H, Heineman MJ, *et al.* The immune response during the luteal phase of the ovarian cycle: increasing sensitivity of human monocytes to endotoxin. Fertil Steril 2001;76:555-9.

[24]   Marino M, Galluzzo P, Ascenzi P. Estrogen signaling multiple pathways to impact gene transcription. Curr Genomics 2006;7:497-508.

[25]   Naugler WE, Sakurai T, Kim S, *et al.* Gender disparity in liver cancer due to sex differences in MyD88-dependent IL-6 production. Science 2007;317:121-4.

[26]   Komi J, Lassila O. Nonsteroidal anti-estrogens inhibit the functional differentiation of human monocyte-derived dendritic cells. Blood 2000;95:2875-82.

[27]   Rachon D, Mysliwska J, Suchecka-Rachon K, *et al.* Effects of oestrogen deprivation on interleukin-6 production by peripheral blood mononuclear cells of postmenopausal women. J Endocrinol 2002;172:387-95.

[28]   Brooks-Asplund EM, Tupper CE, Daun JM, *et al.* Hormonal modulation of interleukin-6, tumor necrosis factor and associated receptor secretion in postmenopausal women. Cytokine 2002;19:193-200.

[29]   Bouman A, Heineman MJ, Faas MM. Sex hormones and the immune response in humans. Hum Reprod Update 2005;11:411-23.

[30]   Loy RA, Loukides JA, Polan ML. Ovarian steroids modulate human monocyte tumor necrosis factor alpha messenger ribonucleic acid levels in cultured human peripheral monocytes. Fertil Steril 1992;58:733-9.

[31]   Konecna L, Yan MS, Miller LE, *et al.* Modulation of IL-6 production during the menstrual cycle *in vivo* and *in vitro*. Brain Behav Immun 2000;14:49-61.

[32]   Schwarz E, Schafer C, Bode JC, Bode C. Influence of the menstrual cycle on the LPS-induced cytokine response of monocytes. Cytokine 2000;12:413-6.

[33]   Rogers A, Eastell R. The effect of 17beta-estradiol on production of cytokines in cultures of peripheral blood. Bone 2001;29:30-4.

[34]   Rachon D, Mysliwska J, Suchecka-Rachon K, *et al.* Effects of oestrogen deprivation on interleukin-6 production by peripheral blood mononuclear cells of postmenopausal women. J Endocrinol 2002;172:387-95.

[35]   Kishihara Y, Hayashi J, Yoshimura E, *et al.* IL-1 beta and TNF-alpha produced by peripheral blood mononuclear cells before and during interferon therapy in patients with chronic hepatitis C. Dig Dis Sci 1996;41:315-21.

[36]   Hsu HY, Chang MH, Ni YH, Lee PI. Cytokine release of peripheral blood mononuclear cells in children with chronic hepatitis B virus infection. J Pediatr Gastroenterol Nutr 1999;29:540-5.

[37]   Gonzalez-Amaro R, Garcia-Monzon C, Garcia-Buey L, *et al.* Induction of tumor necrosis factor alpha production by human hepatocytes in chronic viral hepatitis. J Exp Med 1994;179:841-8.

[38]   Lara-Pezzi E, Majano PL, Gomez-Gonzalo M, *et al.* The hepatitis B virus X protein up-regulates tumor necrosis factor alpha gene expression in hepatocytes. Hepatology 1998;28:1013-21.

[39]   Huang H, He J, Yuan Y, *et al.* Opposing effects of estradiol and progesterone on the oxidative stress-induced production of chemokine and proinflammatory cytokines in murine peritoneal macrophages. J Med Invest 2008;55:133-41.

[40]   McMurray RW, Suwannaroj S, Ndebele K, Jenkins JK. Differential effects of sex steroids on T and B cells: modulation of cell cycle phase distribution, apoptosis and bcl-2 protein levels. Pathobiology 2001;69:44-58.

[41]   Grossman CJ. Regulation of the immune system by sex steroids. Endocr Rev 1984;5:435-55.

[42]   Van Voorhis BJ, Anderson DJ, Hill JA. The effects of RU 486 on immune function and steroid-induced immunosuppression *in vitro*. J Clin Endocrinol Metab 1989;69:1195-9.

[43]   Takao T, Kumagai C, Hisakawa N, *et al.* Effect of 17beta-estradiol on tumor necrosis factor-alpha-induced cytotoxicity in the human peripheral T lymphocytes. J Endocrinol 2005;184:191-7.

[44]   Gilmore W, Weiner LP, Correale J. Effect of estradiol on cytokine secretion by proteolipid protein-specific T cell clones isolated from multiple sclerosis patients and normal control subjects. J Immunol 1997;158:446-51.

[45]   Amadori A, Zamarchi R, De SG, *et al.* Genetic control of the CD4/CD8 T-cell ratio in humans. Nat Med 1995;1:1279-83.

[46]   Cutolo M, Sulli A, Capellino S, *et al.* Sex hormones influence on the immune system: basic and clinical aspects in autoimmunity. Lupus 2004;13:635-8.

[47]   Fagarasan S, Honjo T. T-Independent immune response: new aspects of B cell biology. Science 2000;290:89-92.

[48]   Kasaian MT, Casali P. Autoimmunity-prone B-1 (CD5 B) cells, natural antibodies and self recognition. Autoimmunity 1993;15:315-29.

[49]   Kamada M, Irahara M, Maegawa M, *et al.* B cell subsets in postmenopausal women and the effect of hormone replacement therapy. Maturitas 2001;37:173-9.

[50]   Grimaldi CM, Cleary J, Dagtas AS, *et al.* Estrogen alters thresholds for B cell apoptosis and activation. J Clin Invest 2002;109:1625-33.

[51]   Araneo BA, Dowell T, Diegel M, Daynes RA. Dihydrotestosterone exerts a depressive influence on the production of interleukin-4 (IL-4), IL-5, and gamma-interferon, but not IL-2 by activated murine T cells. Blood 1991;78:688-99.

[52]   Kanda N, Tsuchida T, Tamaki K. Estrogen enhancement of anti-double-stranded DNA antibody and immunoglobulin G production in peripheral blood mononuclear cells from patients with systemic lupus erythematosus. Arthritis Rheum 1999;42:328-37.

[53]   Prieto GA, Rosenstein Y. Oestradiol potentiates the suppressive function of human CD4 CD25 regulatory T cells by promoting their proliferation. Immunology 2006;118:58-65.

[54]   Arruvito L, Sanz M, Banham AH, Fainboim L. Expansion of CD4+CD25+and FOXP3+ regulatory T cells during the follicular phase of the menstrual cycle: implications for human reproduction. J Immunol 2007;178:2572-8.

[55]   Tai P, Wang J, Jin H, *et al.* Induction of regulatory T cells by physiological level estrogen. J Cell Physiol 2008;214:456-64.

CHAPTER 6

Role of IL-6 in Gender Differences of Hepatocarcinogenesis

Hayato Nakagawa[*]

Department of Gastroenterology, University of Tokyo, 7-3-1 Hongo, Bunkyo-ku, Tokyo 113-8655, Japan

Abstract: Regardless of etiology, hepatocellular carcinoma (HCC) develops much more frequently in males than in females in almost all populations. Although sex hormones and X-chromosome-linked genetic factors are considered to be important, the precise mechanism has not yet been elucidated. Recent clinical and experimental studies have revealed that interleukin-6 (IL-6) and the inflammation-mediated signal transduction pathways, including nuclear factor-kappaB (NF-κB), seem to play key roles in the gender difference in hepatocarcinogenesis. In particular, a report by Naugler *et al.* showing that estrogen-mediated inhibition of IL-6 production by Kupffer cells explains the gender disparity in HCC development, gives considerable attention to the association between IL-6 and hepatocarcinogenesis. Investigating the factors causing a gender difference in hepatocarcinogenesis is very important to clarify the carcinogenic pathway and the therapeutic target for HCC.

Keywords: hepatocellular carcinoma, gender difference, sex hormones, liver inflammation, hepatitis virus, interleukin-6, nuclear factor-kappa B, mitogen-activated protein kinase, signal transducer and activator of transcription 3, microRNA.

1. INTRODUCTION

Hepatocellular carcinoma (HCC) is the fifth most common cancer worldwide and the third most common cause of cancer mortality [1]. The age-adjusted incidence rate of HCC varies geographically, being high in East Asia and moderate in Europe, North/South America, and Oceania. Additionally, a definite increase in HCC incidence has recently been reported from Europe and North America. However, the reported incidence of HCC may be underestimated in underdeveloped countries due to insufficient diagnosis or an inadequate registration system [2]. Therefore, understanding the molecular carcinogenic mechanisms and the unique pathogenic biology of HCC has become imperative worldwide.

HCC usually develops after chronic liver damage and often after cirrhosis. Although the etiology of background liver disease varies geographically, chronic hepatitis B virus (HBV) or hepatitis C virus (HCV) is the main cause of HCC in most areas. Other major etiologies include alcoholic hepatitis, hemochromatosis, and non-alcoholic steatohepatitis [1, 3]. During recent years, evidence has been accumulating to show that chronic inflammation has an important role in the initiation, promotion, and progression of HCC. Hepatitis viral-, alcohol-, and hepatic fat accumulation-induced chronic inflammation and the effect of cytokines in the development of fibrosis and liver cell proliferation are some of the major pathogenic mechanisms [4, 5].

A relevant aspect of HCC epidemiology is the gender difference in the incidence of this neoplasm. HCC develops much more frequently in males than in females [1, 6, 7]. This gender difference may be attributable to higher exposure of males to HCC risk factors, such as alcohol consumption and cigarette smoking [3, 8]. However, animal experiments also reveal a higher susceptibility to HCC in males, indicating that the prevalence for HCC in males has a basic molecular basis [9-11]. However, the mechanisms responsible for the gender disparity are largely unknown, although the data suggest that sex hormones such as estrogen and testosterone might be involved in this phenomenon.

Recently, a molecular mechanism explaining the gender difference has been studied in view of the gender difference in immune responses. Naugler *et al.* reported that estrogen-mediated inhibition of interleukin-6 (IL-6) production by Kupffer cells explains the gender disparity in hepatocarcinogenesis using murine HCC

---

*Address correspondence to Hayato Nakagawa: Department of Gastroenterology, University of Tokyo, 7-3-1 Hongo, Bunkyo-ku, Tokyo 113-8655, Japan; Tel: +81-3-3815-5411; Fax: +81-3-3814-0021; E-mail: n-hayato@yf7.so-net.ne.jp

Ichiro Shimizu (Ed)

models [11]. Several reports give considerable attention to the association between IL-6 and hepatocarcinogenesis [6, 7, 12-14]. Hence, in this chapter, I discuss the mechanism of hepatocarcinogenesis focusing on IL-6 and gender differences.

2. INFLAMMATION AND HEPATOCARCINOGENESIS

The development of cancer in various organs is often associated with chronic inflammation, suggesting a strong relationship between inflammation and carcinogenesis [15]. Although first suggested in the 19th century by Virchow, the notion has only become more accepted in the past decade, and molecular mechanisms connecting inflammation and cancer are just beginning to emerge [16]. Abnormal cellular alterations accompanying inflammation, such as oxidative stress, gene mutations, epigenetic changes, and inflammatory cytokine-induced cell proliferation have been proposed as carcinogenic factors [17-19].

Accumulating evidence indicates that a sustained inflammatory reaction in the liver is the major contributing factor to HCC development. For example, in chronic hepatitis C, the host immune responses to HCV are often not strong enough to completely clear the infection, resulting in the chronic stimulation of an antigen-specific immune response [20]. Hepatocyte damage is induced by the continued expression of cytokines and recruitment of activated inflammatory cells to the liver, which is followed by hepatocyte regeneration. This persistent cycle of necro-inflammation and hepatocyte regeneration is thought to provide a mitogenic and mutagenic environment leading to HCC development [5, 21].

2.1. NF-κB

Recently, the signal transduction pathways for inflammation-mediated carcinogenesis have been clarified. A series of high-quality *in vivo* studies strongly implicate nuclear factor-kappaB (NF-κB) as a master regulator of the inflammation–carcinogenesis axis in the liver. The transcription factor NF-κB is a critical regulator of innate and adaptive immune responses, inflammation, and cell survival [22]. Five members, including p65 (RelA), c-Rel, RelB, p50/ NF-κB1, and p52/ NF-κB2 belong to the mammalian NF-κB family and are assembled by dimerization [23]. Without stimulation, most NF-κB dimmers are bound to specific inhibitory factors such as inhibitor of NF-κB (IκB) proteins in the cytoplasm. Many proinflammatory stimuli such as lipopolysaccharide, tumor necrosis factor (TNF)-α, and IL-1α/β can activate NF-κB, mainly through IKK-dependent phosphorylation and degradation of the IκB inhibitory proteins. Stimulation activates the IKK complex, which consists of two catalytic subunits, IKKα and IKKβ, and a regulatory component, IKKγ/NEMO. For most stimuli, IKK activation occurs primarily through IKKβ [24].

Maeda *et al.* demonstrated a critical concept with regard to the different roles of NF-κB in hepatocyte and immune cells using two types of conditional IKKβ knockout mice [25]. They showed that hepatocyte-specific knockout of IKKβ dramatically enhanced chemical procarcinogen diethylnitrosoamine (DEN)-induced HCC. The ablation of hepatocyte IKKβ induces higher DEN-induced c-jun NH$_2$-terminal kinase (JNK) activation and greater cell death during the acute reaction to DEN administration. The absence of NF-κB induces prolonged JNK activation by enhancing reactive oxygen species production, and prolonged JNK activation plays a critical role in hepatocyte death [26, 27]. Subsequently, cell death is accompanied by an inflammatory reaction, and the elevated hepatocyte death rate enhances compensatory proliferation due to the strong regenerative capacity of the liver. Thus, the hepatocyte-specific deletion of IKKβ augments DEN-induced hepatocyte death, cytokine-driven compensatory proliferation, and increased tumorigenesis. Similar findings were obtained in mice lacking IKKγ/NEMO, whose hepatocyte specific deletion results in spontaneous liver damage, hepatosteatosis, fibrosis, and HCC development [28]. On the other hand, mice with IKKβ knockout in both hepatocytes and myeloid cells, including Kupffer cells, have substantially reduced DEN-induced HCC development [25]. This phenotype was associated with markedly reduced hepatic expression of cytokines such as TNF-α, IL-6, and hepatocyte growth factor, which are normally elevated in DEN-treated wild-type mice. These cytokines are secreted by non-parenchymal cells in response to dying hepatocytes and play important roles in compensatory hepatocyte proliferation [29]. These results suggest that IKKβ /NF-κB activation in myeloid cells is important for the production of liver growth factors and subsequent hepatocarcinogenesis. Therefore, IKKβ orchestrates inflammatory crosstalk between hepatocytes and myeloid cells that promote hepatocarcinogenesis. Because pharmacological NF-κB inhibitors are unlikely to be cell-type specific, NF-κB may be potential therapeutic target for preventing liver cancer.

2.2. IL-6

As mentioned above, NF-κB activation-mediated production of inflammatory cytokines in myeloid cells plays an important role in the inflammation–carcinogenesis axis of the liver. Various inflammatory cytokines, including TNF-α, IL-1α, IL-1β, IL-6, and IL-8 have been implicated in chronic liver inflammation, among which IL-6 is thought to be one of the most important [4, 20, 30].

In 1986, Kishimoto and collaborators cloned a DNA encoding a new human interleukin, BCDF/BSF-2, which was later named interleukin-6 (IL-6) [31]. IL-6 is a helical glycoprotein with a molecular weight of 21–28 kD, and its expression is mainly modulated by NF-κB. Under physiological conditions, the main sources of IL-6 are immune cells, vascular endothelial cells, and adipocytes [32]. IL-6 is a potent, pleiotropic, inflammatory cytokine that mediates various kinds of physiological functions such as the developmental differentiation of lymphocytes, cell proliferation, and cell survival. In the liver, IL-6 stimulates hepatocytes to produce a variety of acute-phase proteins, including C-reactive protein, serum amyloid A, complement C3, fibrinogen, and macroglobulin [33]. Recent reports have shown how dysregulation of IL-6 signaling contributes to inflammation-associated disease conditions, including chronic hepatitis, obesity and insulin resistance, inflammatory bowel disease, rheumatoid arthritis, sepsis, and even aging itself [34]. Furthermore, more recent studies have clarified that IL-6 is a key mediator linking inflammation to cancer [35].

Serum IL-6 levels are elevated in patients with chronic liver diseases including alcoholic hepatitis, HBV, HCV infections, and steatohepatitis [36-38]. Furthermore, serum IL-6 levels are reportedly higher in patients with than in those without HCC [39, 40]. Recently, we conducted a retrospective cohort study including 330 patients with chronic hepatitis C to investigate the association between serum IL-6 levels and the risk of future HCC development and found that higher serum IL-6 level was associated with a higher risk of hepatocarcinogenesis [41]. In a case–control study in chronic hepatitis B patients, an association between serum levels of IL-6 and HCC development has also been reported [42]. These findings suggest that IL-6 plays a role linking chronic inflammation and hepatocarcinogenesis in human.

In chronic hepatitis, IL-6, produced mainly by activated Kupffer cells, intensifies local inflammatory responses and induces compensatory hepatocyte proliferation, facilitating malignant transformation of hepatocytes [35]. Hepatocytes express high amounts of the IL-6 receptor and a signal-transducing element gp130, which upon IL-6-binding, activates two signaling pathways, Janus activated kinase–signal transducer and activator of transcription (JAK-STAT) and mitogen-activated protein kinase (MAPK), which are important in the regulation of cell survival and proliferation [43].

2.3. JAK-STAT Signaling Pathway

The JAK-STAT pathway was originally discovered through its capacity to mediate signaling from interferon and IL-6 receptors following engagement with their cognate cytokines [32, 44]. The pathways consist of tyrosine kinase JAKs bound to a group of receptor proteins that demonstrate specificity for each respective cytokine ligand. Cytokines function by specifically recognizing their receptors, which, as a result of binding to their ligand, undergo conformational changes resulting in the displacement of JAKs. Subsequent to the binding of cytokines, JAKs phosphorylate and activate STATs. The activated STAT protein translocates to the nucleus, where it recognizes specific enhancer elements in the promoter and enhancer regions of target genes and initiates transcription.

The STAT protein family consists of seven members, which are encoded by distinct genes: STAT1, STAT2, STAT3, STAT4, STAT6 and the closely related STAT5A and STAT5B [44]. Among them, STAT3 is the most important IL-6 signaling pathway molecule. In response to IL-6 signaling through gp130-JAK, STAT3 forms homodimers that translocate to the nucleus. STAT3 is constitutively active in many tumor cells, but not in normal cells, and regulates the expression of genes involved in tumor progression, such as cell survival genes (survivin, bcl-xL, mcl-1, cellular FLICE-like inhibitory protein) and cell proliferation genes (c-fos, c-myc, cyclin D1) [45]. Additionally, STAT3 interacts with NF-κB at several levels in tumors. For example, STAT3 directly interacts with RelA, trapping it in the nucleus and thereby contributing constitutive NF-κB activation [46]. Furthermore, STAT3 and NF-κB also co-regulate numerous oncogenic and inflammatory genes [47]. Thus, STAT3 and NF-κB play critical roles in inflammation-associated cancer.

Accumulating clinical and experimental evidence has suggested the involvement of the IL-6-gp130-JAK-STAT3 signaling pathway in hepatocarcinogenesis. STAT3 is frequently activated in HCV-infected liver and HCC [48]. He *et al.* reported that 60% of HCC exhibited activated nuclear STAT3 and that STAT3 activation is more pronounced in more aggressive tumors [49]. Suppressors of this pathway, such as suppressor of cytokine signaling 3 (SOCS3), are also downregulated in HCC [48]. Hepatocyte-specific SOCS3 knockout mice enhance their proliferative response during liver regeneration through enhanced activation of JAK-STAT and MAPK signaling and are susceptible to HCC development in DEN-induced HCC models [50]. Hepatocyte-specific IL-6 and IL-6R transgenic mice spontaneously develop hepatocellular hyperplasia and adenomas, which are considered precancerous lesions in humans, accompanying STAT3 activation [51]. Furthermore, in a human study, gain-of-function mutations in gp130, which is the IL-6 signal transducer, was found in 60% of benign hepatocellular adenomas with an inflammatory phenotype and also in a small subset of HCC [52]. Therefore, the IL-6-gp130-JAK-STAT3 signaling axis is an important contributor to HCC development, making it an attractive target for treatment and/or prevention of hepatocarcinogenesis [44].

2.4. Recent Advances in the Role of IL-6 Signaling from Mouse HCC Models

Recently, elegant work conducted by Naugler *et al.* showed that DEN-induced hepatocarcinogenesis is reduced in IL-6 knockout mice, suggesting that IL-6 signaling plays an important role in hepatocarcinogenesis [11]. That study also demonstrated the critical role played by the Toll-like receptor (TLR) adapter protein MyD88 in the production of IL-6 by Kupffer cells. They observed that accumulation of IL-6 mRNA in Kupffer cells incubated with necrotic hepatocytes is markedly reduced in MyD88-deficient mice. Furthermore, deletion of MyD88 suppresses DEN-induced carcinogenesis, indicating that IL-6 production through the TLR-MyD88-NF-κB in Kupffer cells is essential for HCC development. It was suggested that necrotic hepatocytes could act as a ligand triggering TLR-MyD88 signaling and IL-6 synthesis, which promotes compensatory hepatocyte proliferation (Fig. **1**). They also showed in another study that DEN-treated mice exhibit an acute inflammatory response triggered by IL-1α release from necrotic hepatocytes, and IL-1α subsequently induces IL-6 production by Kupffer cells [53]. Indeed, our clinical study revealed that higher serum IL-6 levels correlated with higher AST levels in chronic hepatitis C, suggesting that IL-6 may be produced in response to HCV-induced hepatocyte injury [41]. Furthermore, the risk of HCC development was more strongly associated with serum IL-6 levels than with serum transaminase levels, suggesting a direct relationship between IL-6 and hepatocarcinogenesis in humans.

Several epidemiologic studies have shown that obesity and metabolic syndrome increase the risk of HCC [54, 55]. Although the mechanism by which obesity and metabolic syndrome promote hepatocarcinogenesis is still not fully understood, a recent report by Park *et al.* demonstrated that IL-6 and TNF-α are required for the development of experimental obesity-induced HCC [56]. In obese patients, visceral fat accumulation-induced adipokine dysregulation such as leptin and adiponectin, hepatic fat accumulation, and insulin resistance promote activation of the inflammatory response, which, in turn, increases IL-6 and TNF-α expression by adipose tissue or Kupffer cells. IL-6 and TNF-α activate STAT3 and NF-κB, respectively, which promote cell proliferation of damaged cells through transcriptional activation of genes involved in cell growth and survival. The accumulation of molecular alterations and pathway activation in damaged hepatocytes contributes to HCC development. Hence, IL-6 also has attracted considerable attention as a mediator of the association of obesity with hepatocarcinogenesis [57].

3. GENDER DIFFERENCES IN HCC

Regardless of etiology, HCC develops much more frequently in males than females in almost all populations, with a male-to-female ratio of 2:1 to 4:1, which varies according to disease etiology and geographic region [1, 6, 7]. This gender difference may, in part, be attributable to differences in exposure to lifestyle-related risk factors for HCC, such as alcohol consumption and cigarette smoking [3, 8]. However, sex hormones and X-chromosome-linked genetic factors may also be important because male experimental rats and mice are more susceptible to HCC than are females [9-11]. In fact, male patients with chronic hepatitis C have a higher risk for HCC than female patients even after adjusting for liver fibrosis and alcohol consumption [58]. Furthermore, not only limited to the incidence, this gender difference is also reflected by the poorer prognosis of HCC in males than females [59, 60]. Interestingly, all these advantages for female patients are attenuated after menopause [61], suggesting that female sex hormones may have protective effects on liver disease progression and HCC development.

3.1. Inhibition of IL-6 Production by Estrogen

Investigating the factors causing such gender differences in hepatocarcinogenesis is very important to clarify the critical carcinogenic pathway in HCC. The above-described report by Naugler *et al.* uncovered a molecular mechanism explaining lower HCC susceptibility in females [11].

To investigate the relationship between hepatocarcinogenesis and gender-dependent expression of IL-6, they administered DEN to male and female mice. Although the gender disparity in HCC development is also found in this DEN-induced HCC model, ablation of IL-6 abolished the gender differences in hepatocarcinogenesis, including tumor incidence and survival rate. They showed that DEN administration caused greater increases in serum IL-6 concentration, which could be abrogated by administering estrogen to male mice. High serum IL-6 levels in male mice correlated with higher serum aminotransferases, apoptosis, and hepatocyte proliferation, indicating acute liver damage induced by DEN. The estrogen receptor-α agonist PPT attenuated DEN-induced liver injury in male mice. Ovariectomy of female mice increased serum IL-6, which was prevented by estrogen administration. Although administration of DEN also up-regulates TNF-α mRNA expression, another proinflammatory cytokine thought to be involved in liver regeneration, TNF-α expression did not exhibit gender differences. These results suggest that estrogen-mediated downregulation of IL-6 is critical for the gender differences in HCC development.

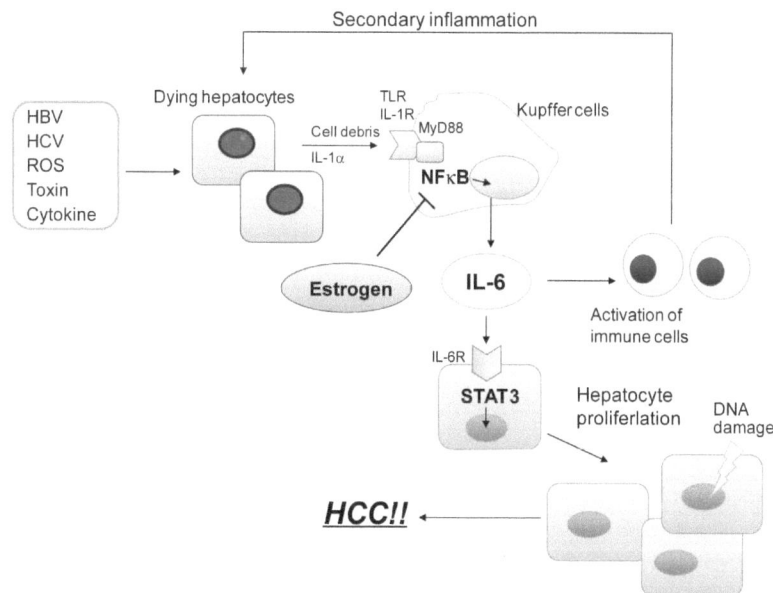

Fig. 1. Current model of the role of interleukin (IL)-6 and the inhibitory effect of estrogen in hepatocarcinogenesis. Dying hepatocytes caused by hepatitis virus, reactive oxygen species (ROS), toxins, and cytokines activate Kupffer cells *via* the Toll-like receptor (TLR) or IL-1R. Activated Kupffer cells secret IL-6 through a nuclear factor (NF)-κB-mediated mechanism. Subsequently, IL-6 induces recruitment of activated inflammatory cells to the liver, which is followed by hepatocyte regeneration. This persistent cycle of necro-inflammation and hepatocyte regeneration provides a mitogenic and mutagenic environment, leading to HCC development. Estrogen inhibits IL-6 secretion from Kupffer cells, which may explain the gender difference in HCC development

IL-6 is mainly secreted by Kupffer cells, so Kupffer cells have been a focus in further investigations of the mechanism of estrogen-mediated downregulation of IL-6 secretion. Kupffer cells from male mice produce IL-6 by incubating them with necrotic hepatocytes in an IKKβ- and MyD88-dependent manner. Interestingly, estrogen administration to Kupffer cells inhibits necrotic hepatocyte-induced IL-6 production. Estrogen inhibits IL-6 promoter activity by decreasing NF-κB and C/EBPβ activity [62]. Hence, estrogen can inhibit IL-6 production by decreasing the MyD88-mediated activation of NF-κB in Kupffer cells. From these results, it was proposed that estrogen-mediated inhibition of IL-6 production by Kupffer cells explains the gender disparity in HCC development (Fig. **1**).

An effect of estrogen is also suggested in humans by the detection of increased serum IL-6 levels after natural and surgical menopause. Furthermore, low-dose estrogen treatment in postmenopausal women causes a reduction in serum IL-6 levels [34, 63].

We have reported that serum IL-6 level is significantly higher in patients with chronic hepatitis C than in healthy subjects and patients with higher serum IL-6 levels have a tendency toward an increased risk of HCC development [41]. This finding supports the important role of IL-6 signaling in hepatocarcinogenesis in humans. However, unlike the mouse model, no significant difference in serum IL-6 levels was observed between male and female patients in our study. One possible explanation for this discrepancy is that 80% of female patients were over 50 years of age, which is the mean age of menopause in Japan, so the inhibitory effect of estrogen on IL-6 production was diminished in most female patients. Indeed, serum IL-6 level tended to be negatively correlated with serum estradiol level in female patients with chronic hepatitis C. Moreover, a higher serum IL-6 level is more strongly correlated with HCC development in female than in male patients. These findings suggest that postmenopausal women have gradually lost the advantage with respect to avoiding HCC development due to the attenuation of estrogen-mediated inhibition of IL-6 production.

3.2. Gender Difference in microRNA Expression

The identification of small, noncoding RNAs in the early 1990s has led to the development of a new research area. Several different classes of noncoding RNAs have been discovered in mammalian cells. These include small interfering RNAs, small nucleolar RNAs, and microRNAs (miRNAs). miRNAs are endogenous 20–23 nucleotides that play important gene-regulatory roles in animals and plants by pairing with the messenger RNAs (mRNAs) of protein-coding genes to direct their post-translational repression [64]. The biogenesis of miRNAs involves a complex protein system including members of the argonaute family, Pol II-dependent transcription, and the RNase IIIs Drosha and Dicer [65, 66].

miRNAs have been recognized to not only regulate normal cell development, but also play an important role in cancer development [67, 68]. miRNAs are frequently located at sites of chromosomal instability or amplification and can act as oncogenes or as tumor-suppressor genes. The most abundant miRNA currently known in the liver, miR-122, is involved in a variety of liver diseases including HCC [69]. miR-122 is significantly and specifically downregulated in rodent and human HCC. Among putative target genes, *N-myc*, downregulated in liver malignancy (*DRLM*), and *cyclin G1* are implicated in hepatocarcinogenesis [70-72]. Among the other miRNAs, miR-21 is highly overexpressed in HCC [73]. Inhibition of miR-21 in cultured HCC cells increases expression of PTEN, one of the most important tumor suppressors in HCC, and decreases tumor cell proliferation, migration, and invasion. In contrast, enhanced miR-21 expression shows the opposite effect. Thus, miR-21 dysregulation is involved in hepatocarcinogenesis through modulation of PTEN expression.

Most recently, Ji *et al.* showed the involvement of miRNA in the gender difference in hepatocarcinogenesis using human samples [74]. They profiled miRNA expression patterns in three separate cohorts of patients with HCC. They found that miR-26 was significantly reduced in HCC tissues compared with surrounding nontumor liver tissues and was more highly expressed in the livers of women than of men. Patients with reduced miR-26 expression had significantly reduced survival during a 6-year period and were more likely to have a response to interferon therapy. Furthermore, mRNA microarray analysis indicated that tumors with reduced miR-26 expression had a distinct expression pattern, and a gene network analysis revealed that activation of signaling pathways between NF-κB and IL-6 might play a role in HCC development (IL-6 expression was inversely correlated with miR-26 expression). Although a causal relationship between miR-26 and hepatocarcinogenesis could not be evaluated in this work, Kota *et al.*, using myc-induced mouse HCC model, reported that low miR-26 expression has a causal role in HCC formation, and replacing miR-26 in HCC with the use of gene therapy could have an antitumor effect [75]. Thus, miRNAs receive much attention not only as oncogenes, biomarkers, and therapeutic targets, but also as causative substances for a gender difference in hepatocarcinogenesis.

4. CONCLUSION

According to recent clinical and experimental studies, IL-6 and the inflammation-mediated signal transduction pathways, including NF-κB, seem to play key roles in the gender difference in hepatocarcinogenesis. Although several factors such as estrogen and miRNAs may be involved in regulating IL-6 expression, the precise mechanism is not fully understood. Because investigating the factors causing the gender difference in hepatocarcinogenesis is very important to clarify the critical carcinogenic pathway and the therapeutic target for HCC, further studies should focus on the details of mechanisms regulating this process.

REFERENCES

[1]   El-Serag HB, Rudolph KL. Hepatocellular carcinoma: epidemiology and molecular carcinogenesis. Gastroenterology 2007 ;132:2557-76.

[2]   Masuzaki R, Yoshida H, Tateishi R, *et al.* Hepatocellular carcinoma in viral hepatitis: improving standard therapy. Best Pract Res Clin Gastroenterol 2008;22:1137-51.

[3]   Yu MC, Yuan JM. Environmental factors and risk for hepatocellular carcinoma. Gastroenterology 2004;127(5 Suppl 1):S72-8.

[4]   Berasain C, Castillo J, Perugorria MJ, *et al.* Inflammation and liver cancer: new molecular links. Ann N Y Acad Sci 2009;1155:206-21.

[5]   Levrero M. Viral hepatitis and liver cancer: the case of hepatitis C. Oncogene 2006;25:3834-47.

[6]   Yeh SH, Chen PJ. Gender disparity of hepatocellular carcinoma: the roles of sex hormones. Oncology 2010;78(Suppl 1):172-9.

[7]   Ruggieri A, Barbati C, Malorni W. Cellular and molecular mechanisms involved in hepatocellular carcinoma gender disparity. Int J Cancer 2010;127:499-504.

[8]   Yu MW, Hsu FC, Sheen IS, *et al.* Prospective study of hepatocellular carcinoma and liver cirrhosis in asymptomatic chronic hepatitis B virus carriers. Am J Epidemiol 1997;145:1039-47.

[9]   Moriya K, Fujie H, Shintani Y, *et al.* The core protein of hepatitis C virus induces hepatocellular carcinoma in transgenic mice. Nat Med 1998;4:1065-7.

[10]   Horie Y, Suzuki A, Kataoka E, *et al.* Hepatocyte-specific Pten deficiency results in steatohepatitis and hepatocellular carcinomas. J Clin Invest 2004;113:1774-83.

[11]   Naugler WE, Sakurai T, Kim S, *et al.* Gender disparity in liver cancer due to sex differences in MyD88-dependent IL-6 production. Science 2007;317:121-4.

[12]   Wands J. Hepatocellular carcinoma and sex. N Engl J Med 2007;357:1974-6.

[13]   Sander LE, Trautwein C, Licdtke C. Is interleukin-6 a gender-specific risk factor for liver cancer? Hepatology 2007;46:1304-5.

[14]   Prieto J. Inflammation, HCC and sex: IL-6 in the centre of the triangle. J Hepatol 2008;48:380-1.

[15]   Shacter E, Weitzman SA. Chronic inflammation and cancer. Oncology (Williston Park) 2002;16:217-26.

[16]   Balkwill F, Mantovani A. Inflammation and cancer: back to Virchow? Lancet 2001;357:539-45.

[17]   Coussens LM, Werb Z. Inflammation and cancer. Nature 2002;420(6917):860-7.

[18]   Maeda S, Omata M. Inflammation and cancer: role of nuclear factor-kappaB activation. Cancer Sci 2008;99:836-42.

[19]   Grivennikov SI, Greten FR, Karin M. Immunity, inflammation, and cancer. Cell 2010;140:883-99.

[20]   Budhu A, Wang XW. The role of cytokines in hepatocellular carcinoma. J Leukoc Biol 2006;80:1197-213.

[21]   Elsharkawy AM, Mann DA. Nuclear factor-kappaB and the hepatic inflammation-fibrosis-cancer axis. Hepatology 2007;46:590-7.

[22]   Karin M, Lin A. NF-kappaB at the crossroads of life and death. Nat Immunol 2002;3:221-7.

[23]   Hoffmann A, Baltimore D. Circuitry of nuclear factor kappaB signaling. Immunol Rev 2006;210:171-86.

[24]   Ghosh S, Karin M. Missing pieces in the NF-kappaB puzzle. Cell 2002;109 (Suppl):S81-96.

[25]   Maeda S, Kamata H, Luo JL, *et al.* IKKbeta couples hepatocyte death to cytokine-driven compensatory proliferation that promotes chemical hepatocarcinogenesis. Cell 2005;121:977-90.

[26]   Kamata H, Honda S, Maeda S, *et al.* Reactive oxygen species promote TNFalpha-induced death and sustained JNK activation by inhibiting MAP kinase phosphatases. Cell 2005;120:649-61.

[27]   Nakagawa H, Maeda S, Hikiba Y, *et al.* Deletion of apoptosis signal-regulating kinase 1 attenuates acetaminophen-induced liver injury by inhibiting c-Jun N-terminal kinase activation. Gastroenterology 2008;135:1311-21.

[28]   Luedde T, Beraza N, Kotsikoris V, *et al.* Deletion of NEMO/IKKgamma in liver parenchymal cells causes steatohepatitis and hepatocellular carcinoma. Cancer Cell 2007;11:119-32.

[29]   Fausto N. Liver regeneration. J Hepatol 2000;32(1 Suppl):19-31.

[30]   Sun B, Karin M. NF-kappaB signaling, liver disease and hepatoprotective agents. Oncogene 2008;27:6228-44.

[31]   Hirano T, Yasukawa K, Harada H, *et al.* Complementary DNA for a novel human interleukin (BSF-2) that induces B lymphocytes to produce immunoglobulin. Nature 1986;324:73-76

[32]   Hodge DR, Hurt EM, Farrar WL. The role of IL-6 and STAT3 in inflammation and cancer. Eur J Cancer 2005;41:2502-12.

[33]   Ramadori G, Christ B. Cytokines and the hepatic acute-phase response. Semin Liver Dis 1999;19:141-55.

[34]   Maggio M, Guralnik JM, Longo DL, Ferrucci L. Interleukin-6 in aging and chronic disease: a magnificent pathway. J Gerontol A Biol Sci Med Sci 2006;61:575-84.

[35]   Naugler WE, Karin M. The wolf in sheep's clothing: the role of interleukin-6 in immunity, inflammation and cancer. Trends Mol Med 2008;14:109-19.

[36]   Deviere J, Content J, Denys C, Vandenbussche P, Schandene L, Wybran J, *et al.* High interleukin-6 serum levels and increased production by leucocytes in alcoholic liver cirrhosis. Correlation with IgA serum levels and lymphokines production. Clin Exp Immunol 1989;77:221-5.

[37]   Lee Y, Park US, Choi I, *et al.* Human interleukin 6 gene is activated by hepatitis B virus-X protein in human hepatoma cells. Clin Cancer Res 1998;4:1711-7.

[38]   Wieckowska A, Papouchado BG, Li Z, *et al.* Increased hepatic and circulating interleukin-6 levels in human nonalcoholic steatohepatitis. Am J Gastroenterol 2008;103:1372-9.

[39]   Soresi M, Giannitrapani L, D'Antona F, *et al.* Interleukin-6 and its soluble receptor in patients with liver cirrhosis and hepatocellular carcinoma. World J Gastroenterol 2006;12:2563-8.

[40]   Porta C, De Amici M, Quaglini S, *et al.* Circulating interleukin-6 as a tumor marker for hepatocellular carcinoma. Ann Oncol 2008;19:353-8.

[41]   Nakagawa H, Maeda S, Yoshida H, *et al.* Serum IL-6 levels and the risk for hepatocarcinogenesis in chronic hepatitis C patients: an analysis based on gender differences. Int J Cancer 2009;125:2264-9.

[42]   Wong VW, Yu J, Cheng AS, *et al.* High serum interleukin-6 level predicts future hepatocellular carcinoma development in patients with chronic hepatitis B. Int J Cancer 2009;124:2766-70.

[43]   Gao B. Cytokines, STATs and liver disease. Cell Mol Immunol 2005;2:92-100.

[44]   Yu H, Pardoll D, Jove R. STATs in cancer inflammation and immunity: a leading role for STAT3. Nat Rev Cancer 2009;9:798-809.

[45]   Aggarwal BB, Kunnumakkara AB, Harikumar KB, *et al.* Signal transducer and activator of transcription-3, inflammation, and cancer: how intimate is the relationship? Ann N Y Acad Sci 2009;1171:59-76.

[46]   Lee H, Herrmann A, Deng JH, *et al.* Persistently activated Stat3 maintains constitutive NF-kappaB activity in tumors. Cancer Cell 2009;15:283-93.

[47]   Yu H, Kortylewski M, Pardoll D. Crosstalk between cancer and immune cells: role of STAT3 in the tumour microenvironment. Nat Rev Immunol 2007;7:41-51.

[48]   Ogata H, Kobayashi T, Chinen T, *et al.* Deletion of the SOCS3 gene in liver parenchymal cells promotes hepatitis-induced hepatocarcinogenesis. Gastroenterology 2006;131:179-93.

[49]   He G, Yu GY, Temkin V, *et al.* Hepatocyte IKKbeta/NF-kappaB inhibits tumor promotion and progression by preventing oxidative stress-driven STAT3 activation. Cancer Cell 2010;17:286-97.

[50]   Riehle KJ, Campbell JS, McMahan RS, *et al.* Regulation of liver regeneration and hepatocarcinogenesis by suppressor of cytokine signaling 3. J Exp Med 2008;205:91-103.

[51]   Maione D, Di Carlo E, Li W, *et al.* Coexpression of IL-6 and soluble IL-6R causes nodular regenerative hyperplasia and adenomas of the liver. EMBO J 1998;17:5588-97.

[52]   Rebouissou S, Amessou M, Couchy G, *et al.* Frequent in-frame somatic deletions activate gp130 in inflammatory hepatocellular tumours. Nature 2009;457:200-4.

[53]   Sakurai T, He G, Matsuzawa A, *et al.* Hepatocyte necrosis induced by oxidative stress and IL-1 alpha release mediate carcinogen-induced compensatory proliferation and liver tumorigenesis. Cancer Cell 2008;14:156-65.

[54]   Muto Y, Sato S, Watanabe A, *et al.* Overweight and obesity increase the risk for liver cancer in patients with liver cirrhosis and long-term oral supplementation with branched-chain amino acid granules inhibits liver carcinogenesis in heavier patients with liver cirrhosis. Hepatol Res 2006;35:204-14.

[55]   Ioannou GN, Splan MF, Weiss NS, *et al.* Incidence and predictors of hepatocellular carcinoma in patients with cirrhosis. Clin Gastroenterol Hepatol 2007;5:938-45, 45 e1-4.

[56]   Park EJ, Lee JH, Yu GY, *et al.* Dietary and genetic obesity promote liver inflammation and tumorigenesis by enhancing IL-6 and TNF expression. Cell 2010;140:197-208.

[57]   Toffanin S, Friedman SL, Llovet JM. Obesity, inflammatory signaling, and hepatocellular carcinoma-an enlarging link. Cancer Cell 2010;17:115-7.

[58]   Yoshida H, Shiratori Y, Moriyama M, *et al.* Interferon therapy reduces the risk for hepatocellular carcinoma: national surveillance program of cirrhotic and noncirrhotic patients with chronic hepatitis C in Japan. IHIT Study Group. Inhibition of Hepatocarcinogenesis by Interferon Therapy. Ann Intern Med 1999;131:174-81.

[59]   Ng IO, Ng M, Fan ST. Better survival in women with resected hepatocellular carcinoma is not related to tumor proliferation or expression of hormone receptors. Am J Gastroenterol 1997;92:1355-8.

[60]   Fukuda S, Itamoto T, Amano H, *et al.* Clinicopathologic features of hepatocellular carcinoma patients with compensated cirrhosis surviving more than 10 years after curative hepatectomy. World J Surg 2007;31:345-52.

[61]   Shimizu I, Ito S. Protection of estrogens against the progression of chronic liver disease. Hepatol Res 2007;37:239-47.

[62]   Stein B, Yang MX. Repression of the interleukin-6 promoter by estrogen receptor is mediated by NF-kappa B and C/EBP beta. Mol Cell Biol 1995;15:4971-9.

[63]   Pfeilschifter J, Koditz R, Pfohl M, Schatz H. Changes in proinflammatory cytokine activity after menopause. Endocr Rev 2002;23:90-119.

[64]   Bartel DP. MicroRNAs: target recognition and regulatory functions. Cell 2009;136:215-33.

[65]   Bartel B. MicroRNAs directing siRNA biogenesis. Nat Struct Mol Biol 2005;12:569-71.

[66]   Kim VN. MicroRNA biogenesis: coordinated cropping and dicing. Nat Rev Mol Cell Biol 2005;6:376-85.

[67]   Calin GA, Croce CM. MicroRNA signatures in human cancers. Nat Rev Cancer 2006;6:857-66.

[68]   Lieberman J. Micromanaging cancer. N Engl J Med 2009;361:1500-1.

[69]   Aravalli RN, Steer CJ, Cressman EN. Molecular mechanisms of hepatocellular carcinoma. Hepatology 2008;48:2047-63.

[70]   Harada H, Nagai H, Ezura Y, *et al.* Down-regulation of a novel gene, DRLM, in human liver malignancy from 4q22 that encodes a NAP-like protein. Gene 2002;296:171-7.

[71]   Gramantieri L, Ferracin M, Fornari F, *et al.* Cyclin G1 is a target of miR-122a, a microRNA frequently down-regulated in human hepatocellular carcinoma. Cancer Res 2007;67:6092-9.

[72]   Girard M, Jacquemin E, Munnich A, *et al.* miR-122, a paradigm for the role of microRNAs in the liver. J Hepatol 2008;48:648-56.

[73]   Meng F, Henson R, Wehbe-Janek H, *et al.* MicroRNA-21 regulates expression of the PTEN tumor suppressor gene in human hepatocellular cancer. Gastroenterology 2007;133:647-58.

[74]   Ji J, Shi J, Budhu A, *et al.* MicroRNA expression, survival, and response to interferon in liver cancer. N Engl J Med 2009;361:1437-47.

[75]   Kota J, Chivukula RR, O'Donnell KA, *et al.* Therapeutic microRNA delivery suppresses tumorigenesis in a murine liver cancer model. Cell 2009;137:1005-17.

CHAPTER 7

Estrogen Reduces Hepatic Fibrosis

Tsutoshi Asaki[1], Tomomi Matsumoto[2], Nozomi Suzuki[2], Chiaki Sagara[2], Yui Koizumi[2], Yoshiki Katakura[1], Yosho Fukita[1] and Ichiro Shimizu[1]*

[1]*Department of Gastroenterology and* [2]*Support Center for Medical Sciences, Seirei Yokohama Hospital, 215 Iwai-cho, Hodogaya-ku, Kanagawa 240-8521, Japan*

Abstract: Oxidative stress, such as the generation of reactive oxygen species (ROS), plays a causative role in the development of hepatic fibrosis. Hepatic fibrosis is a complex dynamic process which is mediated by death of liver cells (hepatocytes) and activation of hepatic stellate cells (HSCs). Multivariate analysis with patients with chronic hepatics C showed that the male sex was associated with advanced fibrosis, which was independent of age at the time of a hepatitis C virus (HCV) infection and of alcohol consumption, and that the progression of hepatic fibrosis began to accelerate at 50 years of age, irrespective of the duration of the virus infection. Judging from these data together with the average menopausal age of 50 years, among premenopausal females without either factors of a male sex or an older age, the transition of hepatic fibrosis to the end-stage cirrhosis appears to require a longer time. The principal estrogen secreted by the ovary and the most potent naturally occurring estrogen is estradiol, which is a potent endogenous antioxidant. Estradiol inhibits ROS generation, antioxidant enzyme loss, and hepatocyte death, and it is also able to attenuate oxidative stress-induced transforming growth factor-β (TGF-β) expression and HSC activation, enhancing antifibrotic activity. Whereas another female sex steroid, progesterone acts in opposition to the favorable effects of estradiol. The stimulatory effect of progesterone on TGF-β expression and HSC activation is blocked by estradiol. These findings suggest that estradiol and progesterone affect coordinately processes related to the slow progression of hepatic fibrosis in females.

Keywords: Hepatic fibrosis, oxidative stress, ROS, hepatic stellate cell, estrogen, estradiol, progesterone, antioxidant, TGF-β, menopause, NADH/NADPH oxidases, lipid peroxidation, collagen, estrogen receptor, apoptosis

1. INTRODUCTION

Multivariate analysis with patients with chronic hepatics C showed that the male sex was associated with advanced hepatic fibrosis, which was independent of age at the time of a hepatitis C virus (HCV) infection and of alcohol consumption [1]. The progression of hepatic fibrosis began to accelerate at 50 years of age, irrespective of the duration of the virus infection [1]. Patients aged over 50 years are reported to have a progression rate of hepatic fibrosis twice as high as those less than 50 years of age [2]. Hepatic fibrosis is a complex dynamic process which is mediated by death of liver cells (hepatocytes) and activation of hepatic stellate cells (HSCs) (Fig. **1**). Judging from these data together with the average menopausal age of 50 years, among premenopausal female persons without either factors of a male sex and an older age, the transition of hepatic fibrosis to the end-stage cirrhosis appears to require the longer time. Indeed, in female patients with hepatitis C, the progression of hepatic fibrosis increases rapidly at menopause. Estrogens include estradiol, estrone and estriol. The principal estrogen secreted by the ovary and the most potent naturally occurring estrogen is estradiol.

At the cellular levels, origin of hepatic fibrosis is initiated by the damage of hepatocytes, followed by the accumulation of neutrophils and macrophages including Kupffer cells (hepatic resident macrophages) on the sites of injury and inflammation in the liver. When hepatocytes are continuously damaged, leading to cell death, extracellular matrix proteins such as collagens predominates are produced over hepatocellular regeneration principally by cells known as HSCs. HSCs are located in the space of Disse in close contact

Address correspondence to Ichiro Shimizu: Department of Gastroenterology, Seirei Yokohama Hospital, 215 Iwai-cho, Hodogaya-ku, Yokohama, Kanagawa 240-8521, Japan; Tel: +81-45-715-3111; Fax: +81-45-715-3387; E-mail: ichiro.shimizu@showaclinic.jp

with hepatocytes and sinusoidal endothelial cells. Their three-dimensional structure consists of the cell body and several long and branching cytoplasmic processes [3]. General structure of an HSC and the space of Disse is represented in Fig. **1**. Overproduced collagens are deposited in injured areas instead of destroyed hepatocytes. In other words, hepatic fibrosis is fibrous scarring of the liver in which excessive collagens build up along with the duration and extent of persistence of liver injury. The trigger is oxidative stress. Hepatic fibrosis itself causes no symptoms but can lead to the end-stage cirrhosis. In cirrhosis the failure to properly replace destroyed hepatocytes and the excessive collagen deposition to distort blood flow through the liver (portal hypertension) result in severe liver dysfunction. Cirrhosis is an important host-related risk factor for the development of hepatocellular carcinoma (HCC) in chronic hepatitis C and B. Staging of chronic liver disease by assessment of hepatic fibrosis always is a major function of prognostic interpretation of individual data including liver biopsy. Of the commonly used staging systems, the METAVIR fibrosis score has been widely used [4]. The stages are determined by both the quantity and location of the fibrosis. With this score, F0 represents no fibrosis; F1 (mild fibrosis), portal fibrosis without septa; F2 (moderate fibrosis), portal fibrous and few septa; F3 (severe fibrosis), numerous septa without cirrhosis; and F4, cirrhosis (Fig. **2**).

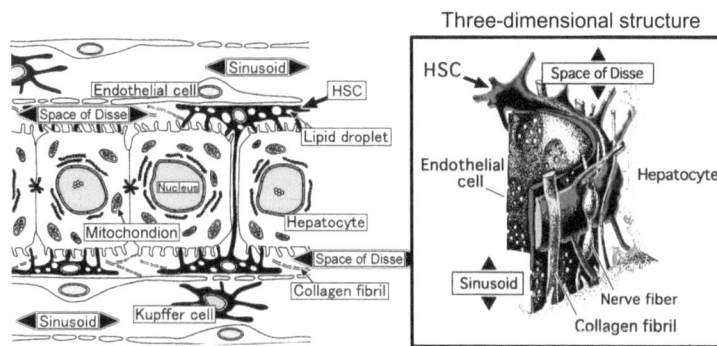

Fig. 1.   Schema of the sinusoidal wall of the liver. Schematic representation of hepatic stellate cells (HSCs) was based on the studies by Wake [3]. Kupffer cells (hepatic resident macrophages) rest on fenestrated endothelial cells. HSCs are located in the space of Disse in close contact with endothelial cells and hepatocytes, functioning as the primary retinoid storage area. Collagen fibrils course through the space of Disse between endothelial cells and the cords of hepatocytes.

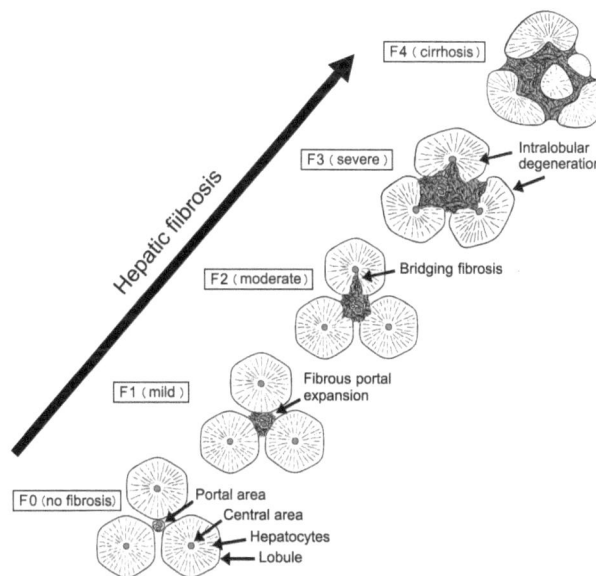

Fig. 2.   Stages of hepatic fibrosis in chronic hepatitis according to the five stages (0-4) of the METAVIR scoring system [80]. With this score, F0 represents no fibrosis; F1 (mild fibrosis), fibrous expansion of portal areas without septa; F2 (moderate fibrosis), fibrous septa extend to form bridges between adjacent vascular structures, both portal to portal and portal to central, occasional bridges; F3 (severe fibrosis), numerous bridges or septa without cirrhosis; and F4 (cirrhosis), the tissue is eventually composed of nodules surrounded completely by fibrosis.

Estradiol is a potent endogenous antioxidant [5]. Hepatic estrogen receptors mediate estrogen action in the liver. This Chapter summarizes the current knowledge of the biological functions of estrogens and the estrogen receptor status as it relates to hepatic fibrogenesis.

2. OXIDATIVE STRESS

Damage of any etiology, such as HCV or hepatitis B virus (HBV) infection, heavy alcohol intake, or iron overload, to hepatocytes can produce oxygen-derived free radicals and other reactive oxygen species (ROS) derived from lipid peroxidative processes [6]. Persistent production of ROS constitutes a general feature of a sustained inflammatory response and liver injury, once antioxidant mechanisms have been depleted. The major source of ROS production in hepatocytes is NADH and NADPH oxidases (respiratory chain-linked enzymes) localized in mitochondria (Table 1). NADH and NADPH oxidases leak ROS as part of its operation. Kupffer cells, infiltrating inflammatory cells such as macrophages and neutrophils, and HSCs also produce ROS in the injured liver. ROS include the free radicals superoxide (O_2^-) and hydroxyl radical (HO^-) and non-radicals such as hydrogen peroxide (H_2O_2). A number of reactive nitrogen species including nitric oxide (NO) and peroxynitrite ($ONOO^-$) are also kinds of ROS. Superoxide production is mediated mainly by NADH oxidase. Hydrogen peroxide is more stable and membrane permeable in comparison to other ROS. Thus, hydrogen peroxide plays an important role in the intracellular signaling under physiological conditions. With respect to pathological actions, ROS participate in the development of liver disease. In this regard, hydrogen peroxide is converted into the hydroxyl radical, a harmful and highly reactive ROS, in the presence of transition metals such as iron (Fig. 3). The hydroxyl radical is able to induce not only lipid peroxidation in the structure of membrane phospholipids, which results in irreversible modifications of cell membrane structure and function (membrane injury), but DNA cleavage (DNA injury) as well. Such a chain of events due to increased ROS production exceeding cellular antioxidant defense systems are called oxidative stress, inducing cell death.

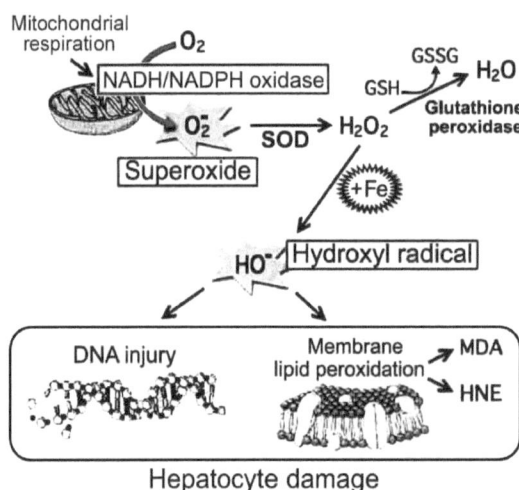

Fig. 3. Oxidative stress and hepatocyte damage [81]. A primary source of reactive oxygen species (ROS) production is mitochondrial NADH/NADPH oxidase. Hydrogen peroxide (H_2O_2) is converted to a highly reactive ROS, the hydroxyl radical, in the presence of iron (+Fe). The hydroxyl radical induces DNA cleavage and lipid peroxidation in the structure of membrane phospholipids, leading to cell death and discharge of products of lipid peroxidation, malondialdehyde (MDA) and 4-hydroxynonenal (HNE) into the space of Disse. Cells have comprehensive antioxidant protective systems, including SOD, glutathione peroxidase and glutathione (GSH). Upon oxidation, GSH forms glutathione disulfide (GSSG).

Malondialdehyde (MDA) and 4-hydroxynonenal (HNE), end products of lipid peroxidation, are discharged from destroyed hepatocytes into the space of Disse. Cells are well equipped to neutralize the effects of ROS by virtue of a series of the antioxidant protective systems, including superoxide dismutase (SOD), glutathione peroxidase, glutathione, and thioredoxin. A single liver injury eventually results in an almost complete resolution, but the persistence of the original insult causes a prolonged activation of tissue repair mechanisms, thereby leading to hepatic fibrosis rather than to effective tissue repair. Hepatic fibrosis, or the excessive collagen deposition in the liver, is associated with oxidative stimuli and cell death. Cell death is a consequence of severe liver damage that occurs in many patients with chronic liver disease, regardless of the etiology such as HCV/HBV infection, heavy alcohol intake, and iron overload.

Table 1. Reactive oxygen species (ROS) production in the injured liver

Major source	mitochondrial NADH and NADPH oxidases (respiratory chain-linked enzymes)
Major producing cells	hepatocytes, Kupffer cells (hepatic resident macrophages), HSCs, infiltrating macrophages and neutrophils
Major ROS family	superoxide, hydrogen peroxide, hydroxyl radical, nitric oxide, peroxynitrite, malondialdehyde (MDA)[a] and 4-hydroxynonenal (HNE)[a] of products of lipid peroxidation
Major antioxidants	superoxide dismutase (SOD), glutathione peroxidase, glutathione, thioredoxin, estradiol

[a]Note the similar characteristics to other ROS.

3. HSCs AND HEPATIC FIBROSIS

Normal liver has a connective tissue matrix which includes collagen type IV (non-fibrillary), glycoproteins such as fibronectin and laminin, and proteoglycans such as heparan sulphate. These comprise the low density basement membrane in the space of Disse. Following liver injury there is a 3- to 8-fold increase in the extracellular matrix which is of a high density interstitial type, containing fibril-forming collagens (types 1 and III) as well as fibronectin, hyaluronic acid and proteoglycans. Collagen types 1 and III are major components of the extracellular matrix, which is principally produced by HSCs. In the resting liver, HSCs have intracellular droplets containing retinoids. Retinoids refer to a group of chemical compound associated with vitamin A. HSCs contain approximately 50-80% of the whole body stores of retinoids [7]. In contrast, in the injured liver, HSCs are regarded as the primary target cells for inflammatory and oxidative stimuli, and they are proliferated, enlarged and transformed into myofibroblast-like cells. These HSCs are referred to as activated cells and are responsible for the overproduction of collagens during hepatic fibrosis to cirrhosis. This activation is accompanied by a loss of cellular retinoids, and the synthesis of α-smooth muscle actin (α-SMA), and large quantities of the major components of the extracellular matrix including collagen types I, III, and IV, fibronectin, laminin and proteoglycans. α-SMA is produced by activated HSCs (myofibroblast-like cells) but not by resting (quiescent) HSCs, thereby a marker of HSC activation. Moreover, activated HSCs produce ROS and transforming growth factor-β (TGF-β) (Fig. 4). TGF-β is a major fibrogenic cytokine, regulating the production, degradation and accumulation of the extracellular matrix in hepatic fibrosis. TGF-β expression correlates with the extent of hepatic fibrosis [8]. This cytokine induces its own expression in activated HSCs, thereby creating a self-perpetuating cycle of events, referred to as an autocrine loop. TGF-β is also released in a paracrine manner from Kupffer cells, endothelial cells, and infiltrating inflammatory cells following liver injury. Similarly, ROS are produced by activated HSCs in response to ROS released from adjacent cells such as destroyed hepatocytes and activated Kupffer cells.

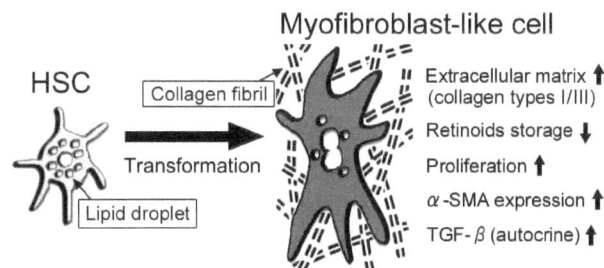

Fig. 4. During liver injury, HSCs are proliferated, enlarged and transformed into myofibroblast-like cells [23]. These activated HSCs produce large quantities of collagens, α-smooth muscle actin (α-SMA), ROS, and transforming growth factor-β (TGF-β), and lose cellular retinoids.

HSCs are activated mainly by ROS, products of lipid peroxidation (MDA and HNE) [9,10], and TGF-β, which are released from destroyed hepatocytes, activated Kupffer cells and infiltrating macrophages and neutrophils in the injured liver (Fig. **5**). In addition to ROS, exogenous TGF-β increases the production of ROS, particularly hydrogen peroxide, by HSCs, whereas the addition of hydrogen peroxide induces ROS and TGF-β production and secretion by HSCs [11]. This so-called autocrine loop of ROS by HSCs is regarded as mechanism corresponding to the autocrine loop of TGF-β which HSCs produce in response to this cytokine with an increased collagen expression in the injured liver [12].

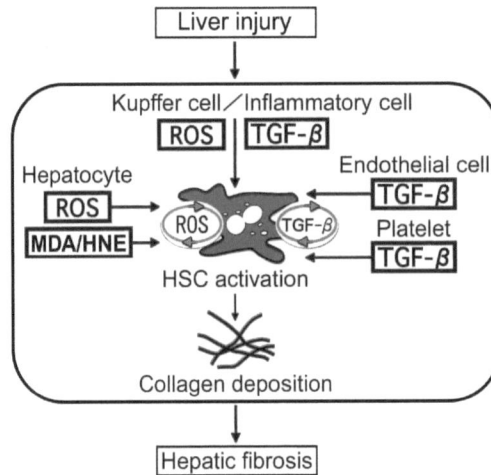

Fig. 5. Activation of HSCs. HSCs are activated by such factors as ROS, lipid peroxidation products (MDA and HNE), and TGF-β released when adjacent cells including hepatocyte, Kupffer cells, and endothelial cells are injured. ROS and TGF-β are also produced by HSCs in response to exogenous ROS and TGF-β in an autocrine manner.

Other important factors for HSC activation are platelet-derived growth factor (PDGF) released from platelets, and endothelin-1 from endothelial cells. PDGF is the most potent mitogen. HSCs congregate in the area of injury, through proliferation and migration from elsewhere, in response to the release of PDGF and monocyte chemotactic peptide-1. Monocyte chemotactic peptide-1 is produced by activated Kupffer cells and infiltrating macrophages and neutrophils. The number of activated HSCs also increases after liver injury [13].

4. CAPILLARIZATION OF SINUSOIDS

Activated HSCs (myofibroblast-like cells), but not quiescent HSCs, can expressα-SMA. Thus, activated HSCs show features of smooth muscle and are contractile. Hepatic sinusoidal blood flow is regulated *via* contraction and relaxation of HSCs. The contraction of activated HSCs in response to inflammatory and oxidative stimuli has important implications in the pathogenesis of portal hypertension in cirrhosis [14]. Two vasoregulatory compounds with obvious effects on HSCs, endothelin-1 and nitric oxide, are produced by endothelial cells [15,16]. Endothelin-1 is the most powerful contractile agent besides an inducer of HSC activation. Exogenous nitric oxide prevents endothelin-1-induced contraction as well as causing precontracted cells to relax. HSCs, Kupffer cells and hepatocytes also produce nitric oxide [17]. Portal hypertension in cirrhosis is caused by increased resistance in the hepatic blood vessels. The increased hepatic vascular resistance is associated with endothelial dysfunction, which can be defined as an impairment of endothelium-dependent relaxation in the liver microcirculation, or HSC contraction due to a decrease in the production of nitric oxide in the liver along with a concomitant increase in endothelin-1. In other words, in advanced hepatic fibrosis activated HSCs induce the excessive collagen deposition and the persistent contraction, and distort blood flow through the liver, resulting in portal hypertension with endothelial dysfunction [18].

Endothelial cells have unique and distinct characteristics from any other vascular endothelial cells for their open pores, or sieve-like fenestrae on the cell surface and lack of basement membrane. Being the first contact of hepatic blood circulation, fenestra structure is important for selecting molecules and substances that enter the liver cells and exchange between the sinusoidal lumen and the space of Disse. Because of the fenestrae and the lack of basement membranes, circulating lymphocytes can also contact hepatocytes directly [19]. During the development of hepatic fibrosis to cirrhosis, the number of fenestra in the endothelial cells decreases, and the basement membrane components collagen type IV and lamimin increase and form a basement membrane-like structure within the space of Disse. These changes of sinusoids are called "capillarizaiton" because the altered structure of the sinusoids resembles that of connective tissue capillaries. Capillarizaiton of the sinusoids causes a disturbance in exchanges of many bioactive substances between the sinusoidal blood and hepatocytes across the space of Disse and thereby contributes to the pathogenesis of advanced hepatic fibrosis and cirrhosis (Fig. **6**).

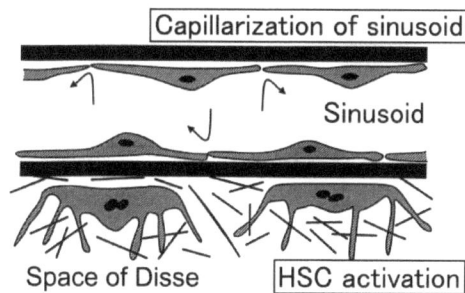

Fig. 6. Capillarizaiton of sinusoids during hepatic fibrosis to cirrhosis. In advanced hepatic fibrosis, endothelial cells themselves acquire a smooth, non-fenestrated surface and a basement membrane-like structure as are found in connective tissue capillaries. These changes of sinusoids are called capillarizaiton.

At the molecular levels, HSCs express the genes which encode for enzymes such as matrix metalloproteinase (MMP)-1 (interstitial collagenase) [20], which digests native fibrillar collagen types I and III, and MMP-2 [21], which digests denatured collagen types I and III and native collagen type IV, as well as tissue inhibitors of MMPs (TIMP)-1 and TIMP-2 [22]. Imbalance between matrix synthesis and degradation plays a major role in hepatic fibrosis [23]. Matrix degradation depends upon the balance between MMPs, TIMPs and converting enzymes (MT1-MMP and stromelysin) [24]. Collagen types I and III constitute the main framework of the so-called "fibrillar matrix". The space of Disse is a virtual space constituted by an extracellular matrix network composed of collagen type IV and non-collagenous components such as laminin. In advanced hepatic fibrosis and cirrhosis, the deposition of extracellular matrix components induces an appearance termed capillarization of the sinusoids as noted above. The large majority of collagen types III and IV, and laminin are synthesized by HSCs and endothelial cells, whereas all cell types synthesize small amounts of collagen type I. During hepatic fibrosis, however, HSCs become the major extracellular matrix producing cell type, with a predominant production of collagen type I [25]. In the resting liver, a balance between matrix synthesis and degradation exists, whereas, in the injured liver, the balance is disrupted. The net result of the changes during hepatocyte damage is increased degradation of the normal basement membrane collagen, and reduced degradation of interstitial-type collagens. The latter can be explained by increased TIMP-1 and TIMP-2 expressions relative to MMP-1. The degradative portion of the remodeling process is coordinated by MMPs and TIMPs.

5. HEPATIC FIBROSIS AND SIGNALING PATHWAYS

Origin of hepatic fibrosis is initiated by the damage of hepatocytes, resulting in the recruitment of inflammatory cells and platelets, and activation of kupffer cells, with subsequent release of cytokines and growth factors. HSCs are the primary target cells for these inflammatory and oxidative stimuli, because during hepatic fibrosis, they undergo an activation process to a myofibroblast-like cell, which represents the major matrix-producing cell. In the injured liver, hydrogen peroxide seems to act as a second messenger to regulate signaling events including mitogen activated protein kinase (MAPK) activation. The MAPK family includes three major subgroups, extracellular signal regulated kinase (ERK), p38 MAPK (p38), and c-Jun N-terminal kinase/stress activated protein kinase (JNK). MAPK participates in the intracellular signaling to: a) induce the gene expression of redox sensitive transcription factors, such as activator protein-1 (AP-1) and nuclear factor κB (NF-κB) [26], b) stimulate apoptosis [27], and c) modulate cell proliferation [28]. ERK and JNK lie upstream of AP-1. JNK and p38 activation are more important in stress responses such as inflammation, which can also activate NF-κB. AP-1 and NF-κB induce the expression of multiple genes involved in inflammation and oxidative stress response, cell death and fibrosis, including proinflammatory cytokines such as tumor necrosis factor-α (TNF-α), interleukin-1 and interleukin-6 and growth factors such as PDGF and TGF-β. TGF-β is a major fibrogenic cytokine, acting as a paracrine and autocrine (from HSCs) mediator as already noted. TGF-β triggers and activates the proliferation, enlargement and transformation of HSCs, but it exerts its inhibitory effect on hepatocyte proliferation [29].

Since many cytokines exert growth factor like activity, in addition to their specific proinflammatory effects, the distinction between cytokines and growth factors is somewhat artificial. No growth factor or cytokine acts independently. The injured liver, predominantly Kupffer cells and infiltrating macrophages and neutrophils, produces TNF-α, interleukin-1 and interleukin-6. These proinflammatory cytokines may also inhibit hepatic regeneration. In particular, TNF-α plays a dichotomous role in the liver, where it not only induces hepatocyte proliferation and liver regeneration but also acts as a mediator of cell death [30]. During TNF-α-induced apoptosis in hepatocytes, hydrogen peroxide is an important mediator of cell death [31].

In liver injury of hepatitis virus infection, transgenic mice expressing HBsAg exhibit the generation of oxidative stress and DNA damage, leading to the progression of hepatic fibrosis and carcinogenesis [32,33]. In addition, HBV X protein changes the mitochondrial transmembrane potential and increases ROS production in the liver [34]. Moreover, structural and non-structural (NS) proteins of HCV are involved in the production of ROS in an infected liver. HCV core protein is associated with increased ROS, decreased intracellular and/or mitochondrial glutathione content, and increased levels of lipid peroxidation products [35]. Glutathione is an antioxidant. NS3 protein of HCV activates NADPH oxidase in Kupffer cells to increase production of ROS, which can exert oxidative stress on nearby cells [36].

6. FEMALE SEX HORMONES ESTRADIOL AND PROGESTERONE

Much of estradiol is converted into estrone and estriol. Estrogens promote development of the secondary sexual characteristics in female individuals and cause uterine growth, thickening of the vaginal mucosa, thinning of the cervical mucosa, and development of the ductular system of the breasts. Estrogens are generated in both females and males, although levels are up to 7-fold higher in premenopausal females than in males and postmenopausal females [37]. Another female sex steroid is progesterone. Progesterone is the principal hormone secreted by the corpus luteum and is responsible for progestational effects, namely, induction of secretory activity in the endometrium of the estrogen-primed uterus in preparation for implantation of the fertilized egg. Progesterone is generated in both females and males, but levels are up to 60-fold higher in premenopausal females than in males and postmenopausal females [37]. Progesterone also induces a decidual reaction in endometrium. Other effects include glandular development of the breasts and increase in basal body temperature. In addition, progesterone has some structural and functional similarities to the principal male sex hormone testosterone [38]. Testosterone is also generated in both sexes, but levels are up to 14-fold higher in males [37]. During the luteal phase of the menstrual cycle in premenopausal females, the blood concentration of progesterone rises up to a maximum of about 10^{-7} mol/L, which is ten to a hundred times higher than that of estradiol [39] (Table **2**).

Table 2. Blood concentrations of estradiol and progesterone in premenopausal female individuals [39]

Sex Steroid Hormone	Phase of Menstrual Cycle	Blood Concentration (10^{-9} mol/L)
Estradiol	Follicular	0.09 - 1.33
	Luteal	0.28 - 0.70
Progesterone	Follicular	1 - 10
	Luteal	28 - 64

7. OPPOSING EFFECTS OF ESTRADIOL AND PROGESTERONE ON HSC ACTIVATION

The female sex hormones estradiol and progesterone have opposing effects on production of ROS and activity of antioxidant enzymes. When production of ROS is enhanced and/or their metabolism by antioxidant enzymes is impaired, a condition called oxidative stress can develop. The production of ROS and decrease of antioxidant enzymes SOD and glutathione peroxidase are inhibited by estradiol, and then they are further stimulated by progesterone both in cultured rat HSCs and human hepatoma cells [12,38]. The major source of ROS production is mitochondrial NADH and NADPH oxidases in the liver. Estradiol inhibits the activation of MAPK intracellular signaling pathways and transcriptional factors of AP-1 and NF-κB *via* the suppression of NADH/NADPH oxidase activity, and inactivates the downstream transcription processes involved in TGF-β expression and HSC proliferation and transformation into the principal matrix-producing cell type [12]. Moreover, TNF-α expression in cultured rat HSCs is inhibited by estradiol. In addition to HSCs, estradiol inhibits the activation of AP-1 and NF-κB in cultured rat hepatocytes in a state of oxidative stress [5,40]. In contrast, progesterone acts in opposition to the favorable effects of estradiol [12] (Fig. **7**).

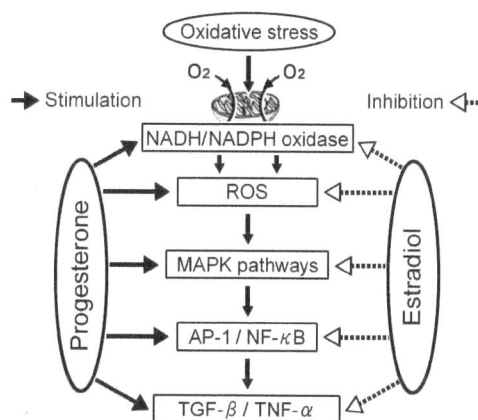

Fig. 7. Estradiol and progesterone have opposing effects on the activation of ROS production processes, MAPK pathways, transcriptional factors of AP-1 and NF-κB, and downstream transcription processes involved in TGF-β and TFN-α in the injured liver [12,38].

The activation processes to α-SMA-positive HSCs, which are regarded as the principal matrix-producing cells, are inhibited by estradiol (Fig. **8**), and are further stimulated by progesterone. Such prooxidative and fibrogenic effects *via* the induction of NADH/NADPH oxidase activity by progesterone are blocked by estradiol at a one hundredth and one tenth dose of progesterone in cultured rat HSCs. These occur at physiological relevant concentration of estradiol (10^{-9} - 10^{-7} mol/L) and progesterone (10^{-8} - 10^{-6} mol/L), equivalent to blood levels of estradiol (10^{-10} - 10^{-8} mol/L) and progesterone (10^{-9} - 10^{-7} mol/L) measured in female persons during their reproductive years [41], and tissue levels of steroid sex hormones may actually be greater [42].

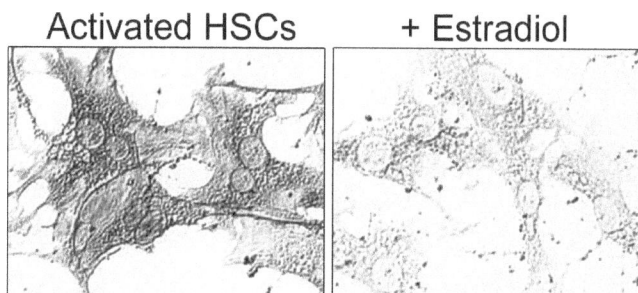

Fig. 8. Estradiol inhibits proliferation, enlargement and transformation of HSCs while progesterone stimulates the HSC activation. Activated rat HSCs are well-spread and positive for α-SMA (Activated HSCs). Estradiol (10^{-7} mol/L) inhibits cell spreading and reduces immunocytochemical staining (darkness) of α-SMA (+ Estradiol).

ROS and TGF-β are produced by HSCs in response to exogenous ROS and TGF-β in an autocrine manner. ROS increase the production of TGF-β and are produced by TGF-β from HSCs, and vice versa. The autocrine loop of ROS and TGF-β in HSCs is prevented by estradiol and induced by progesterone through the regulation of NADH/NADPH oxidase activity (Fig. 9). These data suggest that estradiol and progesterone may work together with the resultant suppression of hepatic fibrosis in female individuals.

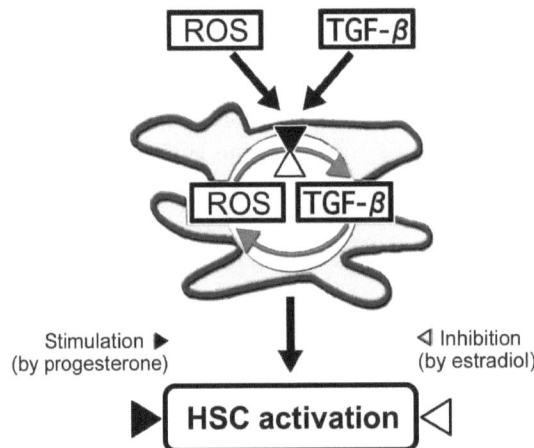

Fig. 9. The autocrine loop of ROS and TGF-β in HSCs is prevented by estradiol and induced by progesterone, leading to inhibition and stimulation of HSC activation, respectively.

8. ESTROGEN RECEPTOR SUBTYPES HAVE DIFFERENT BIOLOGICAL FUNCTIONS

Many of the actions of estradiol are mediated through the estrogen receptor subtypes, estrogen receptor α and estrogen receptor β. The presence of an estrogen binding receptor protein was first reported in the early sixties. An additional estrogen receptor was discovered from animal prostate afterwards in 1996. This novel receptor was designated estrogen receptor β and consequently the originally discovered estrogen receptor was renamed estrogen receptor α [43]. The two receptor subtypes act in distinct ways in several estrogen target cells and tissues [44]. For example, proliferation of the uterus and mammary gland is most likely mediated through estrogen receptor α [45]. Estrogen receptor β exerts antitumoral effects on ovarian cancer cells [46] and plays a protective role against breast cancer development [47]. An interesting difference between the two receptor subtypes is observed on AP-1. AP-1, a transcriptional factor, like NF-κB, induces the expression of multiple genes involved in inflammation and oxidative stress responses, cell death and fibrosis. It is reported that estrogen receptors α and β from an AP-1 site signal in opposite ways when combined with estradiol: with estrogen receptor α, estradiol activates transcription, whereas with estrogen receptor β, estradiol inhibits transcription [48].

Estradiol inhibits activation of AP-1 both in hepatocytes and HSCs. In addition, a high level of expression of estrogen receptor β and a low level of estrogen receptor α expression is seen in human and rat hepatocytes [5,38] and in rat HSCs [49]. Therefore, the inactivation of AP-1 can lead to inhibition of hepatocyte death and HSC activation *via* the reduced expressions of TNF-α and TGF-β when estradiol combined with estrogen receptor β.

9. ESTRADIOL FUNCTIONS AS A POTENT ANTIOXIDANT THROUGH ESTROGEN RECEPTOR

Estradiol and its derivatives are strong endogenous antioxidants that reduce lipid peroxide levels in the liver and blood [50,51]. In hepatocytes besides HSCs and hepatoma cells, estradiol functions as a potent antioxidant [52]. Iron is a strong inducer of the conversion of hydrogen peroxide to hydroxyl radicals in the liver, particularly mitochondria of hepatocytes. The hydroxyl radical can induce not only lipid peroxidation in the structure of membrane phospholipids (membrane injury) but also DNA cleavage (DNA injury), resulting in cell death. Estradiol inhibits the prooxidant iron compound-induced the production of ROS and MDA of an end product of lipid peroxidation, the activation of AP-1 and NF-κB, and the decrease of SOD and glutathione peroxidase activities in cultured rat hepatocytes [5,40]. Estradiol is also able to inhibit the iron-induced lipid peroxidation in isolated rat liver mitochondria [40].

The antioxidant function of estradiol through the endogenous estrogen receptor β is confirmed by using a pure estrogen receptor antagonist ICI 182,780 [53]. Because primary sequences of estrogen receptor β and estrogen receptor α show a high homology in the ligand-binding domain, many ligands show a similar binding affinity for both estrogen receptor subtypes. However, estrogen receptor β and estrogen receptor α have different affinities for and responses to ICI 182,780 [54]. This compound is one of a class of steroidal antiestrogens that bind estrogen receptor with a high affinity similar to that of estradiol and with an estrogen receptor β > estrogen receptor α binding affinity. Thus, ICI 182,780 acts as a pure antiestrogen on both receptor subtypes, particularly estrogen receptor β. ICI 182,780 can block the antioxidant and antifibrogenic functions of estradiol in hepatocytes and in HSCs.

Vascular smooth muscle cells are anatomically analogous to HSCs. Vascular smooth muscle cells express estrogen receptor β at a higher level after vascular injury without significant changes in estrogen receptor α expression [55]. Indeed, the response of arteriolar smooth muscle to injury in some ways resembles that of HSCs [56]. In addition, just like chronic liver disease, atherosclerosis and cardiovascular disease are predominately diseases of male persons and postmenopausal female persons [57]. Several studies document an antifibrogenic effect of estrogens on vascular smooth muscle cells [58,59]. NADPH oxidase is the major source of vascular ROS. Estrogens are reported to lower vascular oxidative stress by modulating the activity of NADPH oxidase and production of ROS, as well as expression of antioxidant enzymes such as SOD [60,61]. Moreover, kidney mesangial cells, which are also analogous to HSCs, have similar properties including playing a prominent role in fibrogenesis. The rate of progression of renal disease is decreased in premenopausal female persons compared with age-matched males. With the onset of menopause and the reduction in estradiol synthesis, the progression of renal disease accelerates [62,63]. Estradiol inhibits the collagen synthesis through estrogen receptor subtypes in mesangial cells [64,65]. These data suggest that estradiol may play the antifibrogenic role mainly through estrogen receptor β in these cells during chronic injury.

In contrast, progesterone can antagonize the vasoprotective antioxidant effects of estradiol [66]. Progesterone enhances NADPH oxidase activity and ROS production, and decreases antioxidant enzyme SOD expression in homogenates of aortic tissues of ovariectomized mice and in vascular smooth muscle cells [60] besides hepatocytes and HSCs. Progesterone interacts with progesterone receptor, which is located in liver cells and HSCs [12,38]   as well as vascular smooth muscle cells [44].

10. ESTRADIOL INHIBITS APOPTOSIS IN HEPATOCYTES

Hepatocyte injury and cell death are a prominent feature of all liver disease processes. Hepatocytes die as a result of either necrosis or apoptosis. The characteristic of necrosis is loss of plasma membrane integrity with release of the cellular contents locally which result in inflammation of surrounding cells and/or tissues. This may potentiate the disease process and lead to further cell death. Apoptosis is the mechanism by which cells self-destruct with the least production of inflammatory response [67]. There are two different reasons why a cell commits suicide through the highly coordinated process:

a) Apoptosis, or programmed cell death, is as necessary for proper development as mitosis is. For example, during embryogenesis excess number of developing cells die and in hormone-responsive tissues, such as the uterus, cyclical depletion of specific hormones leads to death of hormone-dependent cells.

b) Apoptosis is required to destroy cells that represent a threat to the integrity of the organism. For instance, in cells infected with viruses, cytotoxic T lymphocytes target virus-infected cells, inducing apoptosis. Cytoplasm and nucleus/DNA are degraded, eventually breaking into small membrane-wrapped fragments, called apoptotic bodies. Organelles in apoptotic bodies remain viable.

Thus in comparison with necrotic cells, there is minimal release of injurious products, although there may still be fibrotic reaction. Equilibrium within normal tissue depends upon the mitotic rate equaling the rate of apoptosis. Pathological processes can alter the cellular mechanisms involved in apoptosis, leading to liver disease including viral hepatitis B and C and alcoholic liver disease [44,68,69].

During the process of cytotoxic T lymphocyte-mediated apoptosis and necrosis (cytolysis) of target cells, release of lethal hit to virus-infected hepatocytes is mediated by Fas-Fas ligand system and perforin. Cytotoxic T lymphocytes share with other activated T lymphocytes surface expression of Fas ligand, which can deliver apoptosis-inducing signals to target hepatocytes expressing Fas receptor. Activated cytotoxic T lymphocytes recognize viral proteins by the T-cell receptor in the context of major histocompatibility complex (MHC) class I molecules. Binding of Fas ligand to Fas receptor on the virus-infected hepatocytes results in the formation of a death complex, which then activates caspase 8 and triggers the caspase cascade, leading to apoptosis. Caspase 8 activates the protein Bid, which leads to a release of cytochrome c from mitochondria. Cytochrome c also triggers the caspase cascade (caspases 3, 6 and 7) [70]. Apoptosis is blocked by antiapoptotic Bcl-2 family members such as Bcl-2 and Bcl-x_L and promoted by proapoptotic members of this family (Bad, Bak, Bax and so on). In addition, cytotoxic T lymphocytes also release a proinflammatory cytokine TNF-α and cytotoxic granules including a membrane pore-forming protein called perforin after engagement of the T-cell receptor with the viral antigen. Lysis of the hepatocytes is mediated by formation of perforin-induced membrane pores. Binding of TNF-α to TNF receptor on the virus-infected hepatocytes also leads to apoptosis *via* the same pathway as the Fas-Fas ligand system. Therefore, Fas and TNF receptor are called the death receptor.

Oxidative stress is also associated with the Fas-Fas ligand system. In HCV- and HBV-associated chronic liver diseases, lymphocytes infiltrating the liver recognize viral antigens on hepatocytes, become activated and overexpress the Fas ligand on their surface. In alcoholic liver disease, high Fas ligand expression is also observed in hepatocytes. The *de novo* Fas ligand expression is induced by ROS. Parenchymal cell membrane damage results in the release of ROS derived from oxidative stress, which represent a general feature of sustained liver injury of any etiology, once antioxidant mechanisms have been depleted [71]. As hepatocytes also express the Fas receptor, these data imply that hepatocytes may mediate their own death by a paracrine or autocrine mechanism [72].

Viral proteins posses various accessory functions that target host proteins, affecting many signal pathways such as the NF-κB and/or AP-1 pathway. The NF-κB pathway plays an important role in cellular response to a variety of extracellular stimuli, including TNF-α and ROS. NF-κB, in turn, induces the expression of multiple genes involved in inflammation and cell death, such as TNF-α, interleukin-1 and interleukin-6, and TGF-β. TGF-β is produced by HSCs and Kupffer cells and has a dual impact on the progression of liver disease: promoting hepatic fibrosis and killing hepatocytes by apoptosis. Likewise, AP-1 regulates many genes involved in hepatocyte apoptosis and cell proliferation. Both HCV core and HBV X proteins activate NF-κB- and AP-1-associated signals [70].

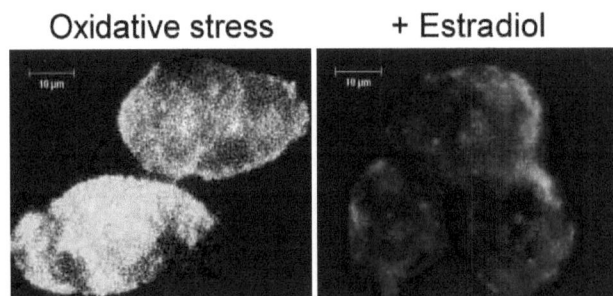

Oxidative stress   **+ Estradiol**

Fig. 10. Estradiol inhibits early apoptosis of hepatocytes in a state of prooxidant-induced oxidative stress [5]. Early apoptosis is detected in rat hepatocytes cultured in the presence of iron compound (Oxidative stress) using fluorescence microscopy. Early apoptotic cells show high white signals, while viable cells show only low signals. Estradiol inhibits iron compound-induced early apoptosis (+ Estradiol).

As shown in Fig. **10**, estradiol prevents early apoptosis of hepatocytes induced by oxidative stress [5]. Prooxidant iron compound and TNF-α are able to induce early apoptosis of hepatocytes *via* the down-regulation of the expression of antiapoptotic proteins Bcl-2 and Bcl-x_L and the overexpresson of the proapoptotic Bad protein [5,38,40]. Estradiol stimulates the expression of Bcl-2 and Bcl-x_L and suppresses Bad expression in oxidative stress- and TNF-α-induced apoptotic hepatocytes. In contrast, progesterone acts in a manner opposite from the inhibitory effects of estradiol on apoptosis of liver cells induced by TNF-α [38].

Judging from these findings and the previous data as above-mentioned, estradiol acts as an endogenous antioxidant and protects hepatocytes from oxidative damage, inflammatory cell injury and cell death by the suppression of NF-κB and AP-1 activation and the induction of Bcl-2 and Bcl-x_L expression, leading to an increase in cellular longevity.

11. ESTRADIOL INHIBITS HEPATIC FIBROSIS

During chronic HCV and HBV infections, hepatic fibrosis eventually reaches the end-stage of cirrhosis, with complications such as HCC. Hepatic fibrosis in chronic hepatitis C and B progresses to cirrhosis more slowly in females than in males [1,73]. Hepatic fibrosis is a complex dynamic process which is mediated by death of hepatocytes and activation of HSCs. As already noted, estradiol is able to inhibit both the hepatocyte death and HSC activation, while progesterone acts in opposition to the favorable effects of estradiol. The stimulatory effect of progesterone on HSC activation is blocked by estradiol at a one hundredth and one tenth dose of progesterone, suggesting that estradiol and progesterone affect coordinately processes related to the slow progression of hepatic fibrosis in female persons.

In *in vivo* studies using animals, estradiol treatment resulted in the inhibition of hepatic fibrosis with a decrease of the number of α-SMA-positive HSCs. α-SMA is an activation marker of HSCs. This was accompanied by a reduced collagen content and lower expression levels of collagen type I and III genes and α-SMA as well as induced expression levels of proapoptotic proteins Bcl-2 and Bcl-x_L in the liver of hepatic fibrosis models in male rats [74-76]. Blocking endogenous activity of estradiol by treatment with a neutralizing antibody against rat estradiol in males and an ovarectomy in females led to enhanced hepatic fibrogenesis [74]. Moreover, estradiol replacement was fibrosuppressive in the castrated females. Another female sex hormone progesterone, however, counteracted the favorable effects of estradiol in a hepatic fibrosis model (Fig. **11**).

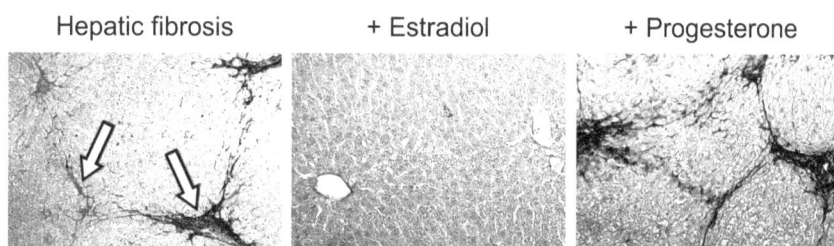

Hepatic fibrosis   + Estradiol   + Progesterone

Fig. 11. Fibrogenesis is suppressed by estradiol and enhanced by progesterone in the liver of a hepatic fibrosis model in male rats. The fibrotic liver has a lot of activated HSCs (arrow) with immunocytochemical staining (darkness) of α-SMA (Hepatic fibrosis). Estradiol reduces the number of α-SMA-positive HSCs (+ Estradiol). Progesterone counteracts the favorable effects of estradiol (+ Progesterone).

Multivariate analysis with patients with chronic hepatics C showed that the male sex was associated with advanced fibrosis, which was independent of age at the time of an HCV infection and of alcohol consumption, and that the progression of fibrosis began to accelerate at 50 years of age, irrespective of the duration of the virus infection [1]. Patients aged over 50 years are also reported to have a progression rate of hepatic fibrosis twice as high as those less than 50 years of age [2]. Judging from these data together with the average menopausal age of 50 years, among premenopausal female persons without either factors of a male sex and an older age, the transition to cirrhosis appears to require the longer time. Indeed, in female patients with hepatitis C, the progression of hepatic fibrosis increases rapidly at menopause [77].

The effect of estrogens on HBV- and HCV-related hepatic fibrosis in humans has rarely been examined. Based on predominantly anecdotal reports, many physicians avoid prescribing hormone replacement therapy to postmenopausal female persons because of concerns regarding potential hepatotoxicity [77]. However, some studies have found that female individuals with lower lifetime exposure to estrogens have an increased rate of hepatic fibrosis progression and that menopausal females receiving hormone replacement therapy present with a lower stage (mild fibrosis) of hepatic fibrosis. Hormone replacement therapy consists of a combination of derivatives of estrogen (transdermic patches or tablets) and progesterone (tablets) [77,78]. These data reinforce the hypothesis of a protective role of estrogens in the progression of hepatic fibrosis.

12. CONCLUSION

Hepatic fibrosis in chronic hepatitis C and B progresses more slowly in females than in males. The menopause is associated with accelerated progression of hepatic fibrosis. Generally, males have a greater opportunity for drinking, and they may fall into alcoholic liver injure easily, although alcoholism is increasing among females, owing to a decline in the social stigma attached to drinking and to the ready availability of alcohol in supermarkets. Factors of social environment and lifestyles may result in a higher preponderance of nutritional and exercise-associated problems in males, and these factors may promote intra-abdominal (visceral) fat accumulation, causing fatty liver in males. Fatty liver histologically results from the deposition of triglycerides *via* the accumulation of fatty acids in hepatocytes, playing a role in the progression of hepatic fibrosis [79].

It could be difficult to clearly distinguish the biological "female sex" factors and the environmental factors in individuals. In practice, both factors are considered to have influence each other mutually, resulting in protection of the female liver from the attacks of inflammatory and oxidative stimuli and cell death. With regard to the female sex factors, estrogens inhibit the ROS production processes and the activation of HSCs, as well as early apoptosis of hepatocytes. These might be leading to reduction of the progression of hepatic fibrosis in females at least.

REFERENCES

[1]   Poynard T, Ratziu V, Charlotte F, *et al.* Rates and risk factors of liver fibrosis progression in patients with chronic hepatitis C. J Hepatol 2001;34:730-9.

[2]   Kage M, Shimamatu K, Nakashima E, *et al.* Long-term evolution of fibrosis from chronic hepatitis to cirrhosis in patients with hepatitis C: morphometric analysis of repeated biopsies. Hepatology 1997;25:1028-31.

[3]   Wake K. Cell-cell organization and functions of 'sinusoids' in liver microcirculation system. J Electron Microsc 1999;48:89-98.

[4]   Huwart L, Sempoux C, Vicaut E, *et al.* Magnetic resonance elastography for the noninvasive staging of liver fibrosis. Gastroenterology 2008;135:32-40.

[5]   Inoue H, Shimizu I, Lu G, *et al.* Idoxifene and estradiol enhance antiapoptotic activity through the estrogen receptor-beta in cultured rat hepatocytes. Dig Dis Sci 2003;48:570-80.

[6]   Poli G. Pathogenesis of liver fibrosis: role of oxidative stress. Mol Aspects Med 2000;21:49-98.

[7]   Blomhoff R, Green MH, Berg T, Norum KR. Transport and storage of vitamin A. Science 1990;250:399-404.

[8]   Castilla A, Prieto J, Fausto N. Transforming growth factors beta 1 and alpha in chronic liver disease. Effects of interferon alfa therapy. N Engl J Med 1991;324:933-40.

[9]   Lee KS, Buck M, Houglum K, Chojkier M. Activation of hepatic stellate cells by TGF alpha and collagen type I is mediated by oxidative stress through c-myb expression. J Clin Invest 1995;96:2461-8.

[10]   Parola M, Pinzani M, Casini A, *et al.* Stimulation of lipid peroxidation or 4-hydroxynonenal treatment increases procollagen (I) gene expression in human liver fat-storing cells. Biochem Biophys Res Commun 1993;194:1044-50.

[11]   De Bleser PJ, Xu G, Rombouts K, *et al.* Glutathione levels discriminate between oxidative stress and transforming growth factor-beta signaling in activated rat hepatic stellate cells. J Biol Chem 1999;274:33881-7.

[12]   Itagaki T, Shimizu I, Cheng X, *et al.* Opposing effects of oestradiol and progesterone on intracellular pathways and activation processes in the oxidative stress induced activation of cultured rat hepatic stellate cells. Gut 2005;54:1782-9.

[13] Enzan H, Himeno H, Iwamura S, *et al.* Immunohistochemical identification of Ito cells and their myofibroblastic transformation in adult human liver. Virchows Arch 1994;424:249-56.

[14] Shimizu I. Impact of estrogens on the progression of liver disease. Liver Int 2003;23:63-9.

[15] Rockey DC, Chung JJ. Inducible nitric oxide synthase in rat hepatic lipocytes and the effect of nitric oxide on lipocyte contractility. J Clin Invest 1995;95:1199-206.

[16] Shah V, Haddad FG, Garcia-Cardena G, *et al.* Liver sinusoidal endothelial cells are responsible for nitric oxide modulation of resistance in the hepatic sinusoids. J Clin Invest 1997;100:2923-30.

[17] Sakamoto M, Ueno T, Nakamura T, *et al.* Improvement of portal hypertension and hepatic blood flow in cirrhotic rats by oestrogen. Eur J Clin Invest 2005;35:220-5.

[18] Iwakiri Y, Groszmann RJ. Vascular endothelial dysfunction in cirrhosis. J Hepatol 2007;46:927-34.

[19] Braet F, Wisse E. Structural and functional aspects of liver sinusoidal endothelial cell fenestrae: a review. Comp Hepatol 2002;1:1.

[20] Casini A, Ceni E, Salzano R, *et al.* Acetaldehyde regulates the gene expression of matrix-metalloproteinase- 1 and -2 in human fat-storing cells. Life Sci 1994;55:1311-6.

[21] Milani S, Herbst H, Schuppan D, *et al.* Differential expression of matrix-metalloproteinase-1 and -2 genes in normal and fibrotic human liver. Am J Pathol 1994;144:528-37.

[22] Iredale JP, Murphy G, Hembry RM, *et al.* Human hepatic lipocytes synthesize tissue inhibitor of metalloproteinases-1. Implications for regulation of matrix degradation in liver. J Clin Invest 1992;90:282-7.

[23] Shimizu I. Antifibrogenic therapies in chronic HCV infection. Curr Drug Targets Infect Disord 2001;1:227-40.

[24] Li D, Friedman SL. Liver fibrogenesis and the role of hepatic stellate cells: new insights and prospects for therapy. J Gastroenterol Hepatol 1999;14:618-33.

[25] Maher JJ, McGuire RF. Extracellular matrix gene expression increases preferentially in rat lipocytes and sinusoidal endothelial cells during hepatic fibrosis *in vivo*. J Clin Invest 1990;86:1641-8.

[26] Pinkus R, Weiner LM, Daniel V. Role of oxidants and antioxidants in the induction of AP-1, NF-kappaB, and glutathione S-transferase gene expression. J Biol Chem 1996;271:13422-9.

[27] Clement MV, Pervaiz S. Reactive oxygen intermediates regulate cellular response to apoptotic stimuli: an hypothesis. Free Radic Res 1999;30:247-52.

[28] Lundberg AS, Hahn WC, Gupta P, Weinberg RA. Genes involved in senescence and immortalization. Curr Opin Cell Biol 2000;12:705-9.

[29] Nakamura T, Tomita Y, Hirai R, *et al.* Inhibitory effect of transforming growth factor-beta on DNA synthesis of adult rat hepatocytes in primary culture. Biochem Biophys Res Commun 1985;133:1042-50.

[30] Schwabe RF, Brenner DA. Mechanisms of Liver Injury. I. TNF-alpha-induced liver injury: role of IKK, JNK, and ROS pathways. Am J Physiol Gastrointest Liver Physiol 2006;290:G583-G589.

[31] Bohler T, Waiser J, Hepburn H, *et al.* TNF-alpha and IL-1alpha induce apoptosis in subconfluent rat mesangial cells. Evidence for the involvement of hydrogen peroxide and lipid peroxidation as second messengers. Cytokine 2000;12:986-91.

[32] Hagen TM, Huang S, Curnutte J, *et al.* Extensive oxidative DNA damage in hepatocytes of transgenic mice with chronic active hepatitis destined to develop hepatocellular carcinoma. Proc Natl Acad Sci U S A 1994;91:12808-12.

[33] Nakamoto Y, Suda T, Momoi T, Kaneko S. Different procarcinogenic potentials of lymphocyte subsets in a transgenic mouse model of chronic hepatitis B. Cancer Res 2004;64:3326-33.

[34] Waris G, Huh KW, Siddiqui A. Mitochondrially associated hepatitis B virus X protein constitutively activates transcription factors STAT-3 and NF-kappa B *via* oxidative stress. Mol Cell Biol 2001;21:7721-30.

[35] Moriya K, Nakagawa K, Santa T, *et al.* Oxidative stress in the absence of inflammation in a mouse model for hepatitis C virus-associated hepatocarcinogenesis. Cancer Res 2001;61:4365-70.

[36] Thoren F, Romero A, Lindh M, *et al.* A hepatitis C virus-encoded, nonstructural protein (NS3) triggers dysfunction and apoptosis in lymphocytes: role of NADPH oxidase-derived oxygen radicals. J Leukoc Biol 2004;76:1180-6.

[37] Czubryt MP, Espira L, Lamoureux L, Abrenica B. The role of sex in cardiac function and disease. Can J Physiol Pharmacol 2006;84:93-109.

[38] Cheng X, Shimizu I, Yuan Y, *et al.* Effects of estradiol and progesterone on tumor necrosis factor alpha-induced apoptosis in human hepatoma HuH-7 cells. Life Sci 2006;79:1988-94.

[39] Clayton RN, Royston JP, Chapman J, *et al.* Is changing hypothalamic activity important for control of ovulation? Br Med J (Clin Res Ed) 1987;295:7-12.

[40] Omoya T, Shimizu I, Zhou Y, *et al.* Effects of idoxifene and estradiol on NF-κB activation in cultured rat hepatocytes undergoing oxidative stress. Liver 2001;21:183-91.

[41] White MM, Zamudio S, Stevens T, *et al.* Estrogen, progesterone, and vascular reactivity: potential cellular mechanisms. Endocr Rev 1995;16:739-51.

[42] Meizel S, Turner KO. Progesterone acts at the plasma membrane of human sperm. Mol Cell Endocrinol 1991;11:R1-R5.

[43] Kuiper GG, Enmark E, Pelto-Huikko M, *et al.* Cloning of a novel receptor expressed in rat prostate and ovary. Proc Natl Acad Sci U S A 1996;93:5925-30.

[44] Hayashi N, Mita E. Involvement of Fas system-mediated apoptosis in pathogenesis of viral hepatitis. J Viral Hepat 1999;6:357-65.

[45] Zhao C, hlman-Wright K, Gustafsson JA. Estrogen receptor beta: an overview and update. Nucl Recept Signal 2008;6:e003.

[46] Treeck O, Pfeiler G, Mitter D, *et al.* Estrogen receptor ?A1 exerts antitumoral effects on SK-OV-3 ovarian cancer cells. J Endocrinol 2007;193:421-33.

[47] Chang EC, Frasor J, Komm B, Katzenellenbogen BS. Impact of estrogen receptor beta on gene networks regulated by estrogen receptor alpha in breast cancer cells. Endocrinology 2006;147:4831-42.

[48] Paech K, Webb P, Kuiper GG, *et al.* Differential ligand activation of estrogen receptors ERalpha and ERbeta at AP1 sites. Science 1997;277:1508-10.

[49] Zhou Y, Shimizu I, Lu G, *et al.* Hepatic stellate cells contain the functional estrogen receptor beta but not the estrogen receptor alpha in male and female rats. Biochem Biophys Res Commun 2001;286:1059-65.

[50] Yoshino K, Komura S, Watanabe I, *et al.* Effect of estrogens on serum and liver lipid peroxide levels in mice. J Clin Biochem Nutr 1987;3:233-9.

[51] Lacort M, Leal AM, Liza M, *et al.* Protective effect of estrogens and catecholestrogens against peroxidative membrane damage *in vitro.* Lipids 1995;30:141-6.

[52] Liu Y, Shimizu I, Omoya T, *et al.* Protective effect of estradiol on hepatocytic oxidative damage. World J Gastroenterol 2002;8:363-6.

[53] Wakeling AE, Bowler J. ICI 182,780, a new antioestrogen with clinical potential. J Steroid Biochem Mol Biol 1992;43:173-7.

[54] Paige LA, Christensen DJ, Gron H, *et al.* Estrogen receptor (ER) modulators each induce distinct conformational changes in ER alpha and ER beta. Proc Natl Acad Sci U S A 1999;96:3999-4004.

[55] Lindner V, Kim SK, Karas RH, *et al.* Increased expression of estrogen receptor-?A mRNA in male blood vessels after vascular injury. Circ Res 1998;83:224-9.

[56] Pinzani M, Failli P, Ruocco C, *et al.* Fat-storing cells as liver-specific pericytes. Spatial dynamics of agonist-stimulated intracellular calcium transients. J Clin Invest 1992;90:642-6.

[57] Vitale C, Miceli M, Rosano GM. Gender-specific characteristics of atherosclerosis in menopausal women: risk factors, clinical course and strategies for prevention. Climacteric 2007;10 Suppl 2:16-20.

[58] Iafrati MD, Karas RH, Aronovitz M, *et al.* Estrogen inhibits the vascular injury response in estrogen receptor alpha-deficient mice. Nat Med 1997;3:545-8.

[59] Bayard F, Clamens S, Meggetto F, *et al.* Estrogen synthesis, estrogen metabolism, and functional estrogen receptors in rat arterial smooth muscle cells in culture. Endocrinology 1995;136:1523-9.

[60] Wassmann K, Wassmann S, Nickenig G. Progesterone antagonizes the vasoprotective effect of estrogen on antioxidant enzyme expression and function. Circ Res 2005;97:1046-54.

[61] Miller AA, De Silva TM, Jackman KA, Sobey CG. Effect of gender and sex hormones on vascular oxidative stress. Clin Exp Pharmacol Physiol 2007;34:1037-43.

[62] Neugarten J, Acharya A, Silbiger SR. Effect of gender on the progression of nondiabetic renal disease: a meta-analysis. J Am Soc Nephrol 2000;11:319-29.

[63] Dubey RK, Zacharia LC, Gillespie DG, *et al.* Catecholamines block the antimitogenic effect of estradiol on human glomerular mesangial cells. Hypertension 2003;42:349-55.

[64] Kwan G, Neugarten J, Sherman M, *et al.* Effects of sex hormones on mesangial cell proliferation and collagen synthesis. Kidney Int 1996;50:1173-9.

[65] Matsuda T, Yamamoto T, Muraguchi A, Saatcioglu F. Cross-talk between transforming growth factor-beta and estrogen receptor signaling through Smad3. J Biol Chem 2001;276:42908-14.

[66] Qiao X, McConnell KR, Khalil RA. Sex steroids and vascular responses in hypertension and aging. Gend Med 2008;5 Suppl A:S46-S64.

[67] Patel T, Steer CJ, Gores GJ. Apoptosis and the liver: A mechanism of disease, growth regulation, and carcinogenesis. Hepatology 1999;30:811-5.

[68] Natori S, Rust C, Stadheim LM, *et al.* Hepatocyte apoptosis is a pathologic feature of human alcoholic hepatitis. J Hepatol 2001;34:248-53.

[69] Guattery JM, Faloon WW, Biery DL. Effect of ethinyl estradiol on chronic active hepatitis [letter] [corrected and republished letter originally printed in Ann Intern Med 1996 Oct 15;125(8):700]. Ann Intern Med 1997;126:88.

[70] Kountouras J, Zavos C, Chatzopoulos D. Apoptosis in hepatitis C. J Viral Hepat 2003;10:335-42.

[71] Houglum K, Filip M, Witztum JL, Chojkier M. Malondialdehyde and 4-hydroxynonenal protein adducts in plasma and liver of rats with iron overload. J Clin Invest 1990;86:1991-8.

[72] Rust C, Gores GJ. Apoptosis and liver disease. Am J Med 2000;108:567-74.

[73] Poynard T, Mathurin P, Lai CL, *et al.* A comparison of fibrosis progression in chronic liver diseases. J Hepatol 2003;38:257-65.

[74] Yasuda M, Shimizu I, Shiba M, Ito S. Suppressive effects of estradiol on dimethylnitrosamine-induced fibrosis of the liver in rats [see comments]. Hepatology 1999;29:719-27.

[75] Shimizu I, Mizobuchi Y, Shiba M, *et al.* Inhibitory effect of estradiol on activation of rat hepatic stellate cells *in vivo* and *in vitro.* Gut 1999;44:127-36.

[76] Lu G, Shimizu I, Cui X, *et al.* Antioxidant and antiapoptotic activities of idoxifene and estradiol in hepatic fibrosis in rats. Life Sci 2004;74:897-907.

[77] Di Martino V, Lebray P, Myers RP, *et al.* Progression of liver fibrosis in women infected with hepatitis C: long-term benefit of estrogen exposure. Hepatology 2004;40:1426-33.

[78] Codes L, Asselah T, Cazals-Hatem D, *et al.* Liver fibrosis in women with chronic hepatitis C: evidence for the negative role of the menopause and steatosis and the potential benefit of hormone replacement therapy. Gut 2007;56:390-5.

[79] Shimizu I, Kohno N, Tamaki K, *et al.* Female hepatology: favorable role of estrogen in chronic liver disease with hepatitis B virus infection. World J Gastroenterol 2007;13:4295-305.

[80] Intraobserver and interobserver variations in liver biopsy interpretation in patients with chronic hepatitis C. The French METAVIR Cooperative Study Group. Hepatology 1994;20:15-20.

[81] Shimizu I, Ito S. Protection of estrogens against the progression of chronic liver disease. Hepatol Res 2007;37:239-47.

CHAPTER 8

Pharmacological Effects of Estrogen in Liver Cirrhosis-Induced Portal Hypertension

Takato Ueno[*]

Research Center for Innovative Cancer Therapy, Kurume University, 67 Asahi-machi, Kurume 830-0011, Japan

Abstract: In the livers of humans, cats, and guinea pigs, nerve endings are distributed all over the hepatic lobules. Nerve endings in the intralobular spaces are localized mainly in the Disse spaces, and are oriented towards the hepatic stellate cells (HSCs), sinusoidal endothelial cells (SECs) and hepatocytes. They are especially closely related to HSCs. Various neurotransmitters such as substance P (SP) exist in the nerve endings. In addition, HSCs possess endothelin (ET) and adrenergic receptors, and contract in response to the corresponding agonists. In contrast, nitric oxide (NO) inhibits the contraction of HSCs. HSCs thus appear to be involved in the regulation of hepatic sinusoidal microcirculation by contraction and relaxation. In the cirrhotic liver, intralobular innervation is decreased, but NO is overexpressed in the SECs. These findings indicate that the sinusoidal microcirculation through NO rather than through intralobular innervation may be involved in cirrhotic liver. Moreover, estrogen plays an important role in the enhancement of NO production in the SECs of cirrhotic liver and reduces the portal pressure.

Keywords: Liver cirrhosis, portal hypertension, estrogen, 17β-estradiol, vascular tone, hepatic stellate cells, hepatic sinusoidal endothelial cells, neurotransmitters, substance P, endothelin, nitric oxide, hepatic blood flow, portal venous pressure.

1. INTRODUCTION

From numerous studies, estrogen is known to be deeply related to various liver diseases. Especially estrogen has antioxidant effect, vascular dilatation, lipid metabolism, and antifibrotic effect in the liver. In this chapter, the relationships between estrogen and the sinusoidal microcirculation in the normal and cirrhotic livers are reviewed and discussed.

2. VASCULAR TONE AND ESTROGEN

Endothelin (ET)-1 and nitric oxide (NO) play important roles in the microcirculation. ET [1] and NO [2] have been identified, and the characteristics of these substances have been determined. ET, which has three isoforms, is a peptide composed of 21 amino acids, and has a potent vasoconstrictive effect on the smooth muscle cells in the vessels. On the other hand, ET receptors were confirmed by the identification and cloning of the ET_A receptor and the ET_B receptor, both of which belong to the superfamily of G protein-coupled receptors [3]. The ET_A receptor binds ET-1 and ET-2 with a higher affinity than ET-3, and the ET_B receptor displays similar affinity for all three isopeptides. The stimulation of ET_A receptors increases the cyclic adenosine 3', 5'-monophosphate (cAMP) level in the cells, while the ET_B receptor is associated with an inhibition of the adenyl cyclase system [4]. In addition, ET_B receptor activates Ca^{2+}-dependent stimulation of constitutive NO synthase [5]. In 1994, the existence of two ET_B receptor subtypes, ET_{B1} and ET_{B2}, has been postulated [6]. ET_A and ET_{B1} receptors induce the contraction of smooth muscle cells, while ET_{B2} receptors of endothelial cells promote vasodilatation through the production of diffusible NO [6, 7].

NO is synthesized from L-arginine by way of NO synthases (NOSs). Three isoforms of NOS have been identified. These are the inducible calcium-dependent isoforms derived from neurons (nNOS or NOS 1) and vascular endothelial cells (eNOS or NOS 3), and a cytokine-inducible calcium-independent isoform (iNOS or NOS 2). Recently, it is reported that NOS localizes in the mitochondria (mtNOS) [8]

*Address correspondence to Takato Ueno: Research Center for Innovative Cancer Therapy, Kurume University, 67 Asahi-machi, Kurume 830-0011, Japan; Tel: +81-942-31-7746; Fax: +81-942-31-7747; E-mail: takato@med.kurume-u.ac.jp

Ichiro Shimizu (Ed)

The relationship between NO and endothelins in the control of vascular tone is physiologically important [9]. Liu, *et al.* [7] reported that ET-1 binding to the ET_B receptor causes eNOS activation *via* Akt phosphorylation, with resultant downstream eNOS phosphorylation and NO synthesis. Furthermore, they found a crucial role for G-protein βγ subunits in the endothelin/NO signaling cascade. The same stimuli that upregulate ET expression and vascular sensitivity to ET also upregulate NOS and heme oxgenase-1. Both catalyze the production of gases that can mediate vasodilatation *via* activation of guanylate cyclase [9, 10].

There is substantial interest in the effects of estrogen on the vascular well, due to the marked gender difference in the incidence of clinically apparent coronary heart disease, when comparing premenopausal women with age-matched males. Recent randomized clinical trials unexpectedly failed to demonstrate a hormone replacement therapy benefit for coronary heart disease secondary or primary prevention in postmenopausal women. There is several possible explanation for these findings, which have created a conundrum in light of the numerous potentially beneficial vascular effects of estrogen demonstrated at the cellular, molecular, and even animal model level. Although estrogen receptors (ERs) are traditionally defined as ligand-activated transcriptional activators or repressors, a phenomenon certainly involved in some of estrogen's beneficial effects on the vascular cells, and the presence of membrane-associated ERs in endothelial cells. The rapid assembly of a membrane-associated molecular complex, comprised of ER, c-Src and the regulatory unit of phosphatidylinositol 3-kinase, p85, in response to estrogen [11].

3. MICROCIRCULATION IN HEPATIC SINUSOIDS

The structure of the sinusoidal wall resembles that of a capillary (Fig. **1**). That is, sinusoidal endothelial cells (SECs) are homologous to capillary endothelial cells, and hepatic stellate cells (HSCs), located in the Disse spaces, are homologous to pericytes located around capillary. The sinusoidal walls organized by SECs, HSCs and so on play important roles in the sinusoidal microcirculation [12, 13]. In the human liver, intralobular nerve endings are located in the Disse space [14-19]. Nerve endings at this site are close to HSCs, SECs and hepatocytes [15-17]. Innervation of the human liver is primarily adrenergic, and some cholinergic innervation is also observed [15, 18, 20-22]. In addition, innervation mediated by various neurotransmitters such as substance P (SP), vasoactive intestinal peptide (VIP), somatostatin, cholecystokinin, neurotensin, amine, NO, calcitonin gene-related peptide and neuropeptide Y has been reported to exist in the human liver [15, 18, 19, 23-25]. We reported that rat HSCs were contracted by ET-1 or SP, and were dilated by NO produced by HSC *via* IL-1 [26, 27]. In addition, we showed that estradiol upregulates NO synthase expression in cultured rat hepatic SECs [28] (Fig. **2**).

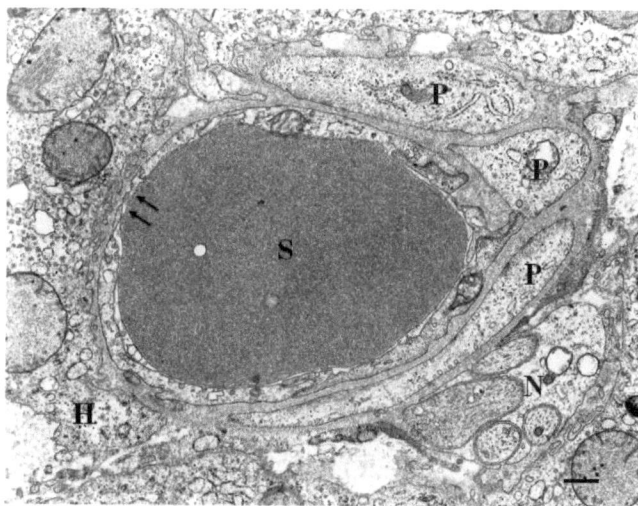

Fig. 1. A transmission electron micrograph showing a hepatic sinusoid in the human normal liver.
Hepatic SECs with fenestrae (arrows) are enfolded by the cytoplasmic processes of HSCs. A naked nerve ending closely faces the process of HSCs.
S: sinusoid, **P**: process of HSCs, **N**: nerve ending, **H**: hepatocyte

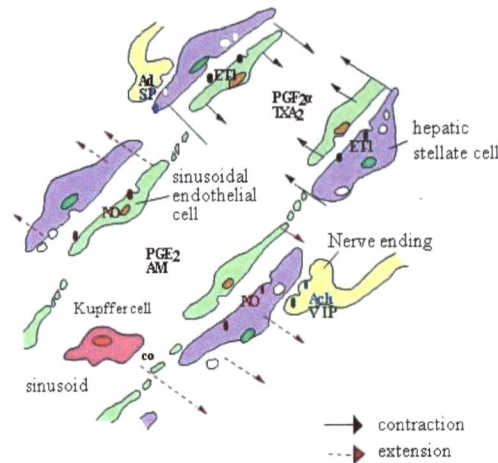

Fig. 2. A diagram showing the relationship between hepatic sinusoidal walls and vasoactive agents in the normal liver. In the normal liver, the sinusoidal microcirculation is suggested to be mainly regulated through the contraction and relaxation of HSCs and SECs by neurotransmitters secreted from nerve endings in the Disse spaces and vasoactive agents such as ET-1, NO and CO.
Ad: adrenalin, **SP**: substance P, **ET-1**: endothelin 1, **PGF**: prostaglandin, **TKA**: thromboxane, **NO**: nitric oxide, **PGE**: prostaglandin, **AM**: adrenomedullin, **Ach**: acetylcholine, **VIP**: vasoactive intestinal peptide, **CO**: carbon monoxide

4. SINUSOIDAL CAPILLARIZATION IN LIVER CIRRHOSIS AND PORTAL HYPERTENSION

Commonly, the thin peripheral portions of SECs are fenestrated, presenting a sieve like appearance. Moreover, the basement membranes, which are visible in capillaries, are hardly seen on the basal side of SECs. In chronic liver diseases such as liver cirrhosis, however, continuous basement membranes are observed on the basal side of SECs, causing hepatic sinusoidal capillarization. In these conditions, SECs show morphological changes resembling the characteristics of vascular endothelial cells: in addition to the formation of basement membranes, the decrease or disappearance of fenestrae and the presence of Weibel-Palade bodies (WPBs) (Fig. **3**), which control the production of factor VIII-related antigen [29]. In addition, liver fibrosis is characterized by the accumulation of extracellular matrix components in the Disse spaces, forming a so-called "capillarization" of the sinusoids. At this stage, resistance in the sinusoidal walls is increased, and the progression of liver fibrosis, intralobular innervation becomes scant, whereas the role of lipocytes in the hepatic sinusoidal microcirculation may become more prominent. In addition, the regulation of these functions in sinusoids of the cirrhotic liver seems to be regulated by agents such as ET-1 and NO in a paracrine or autocrine manner [26, 27] (Fig. **4**).

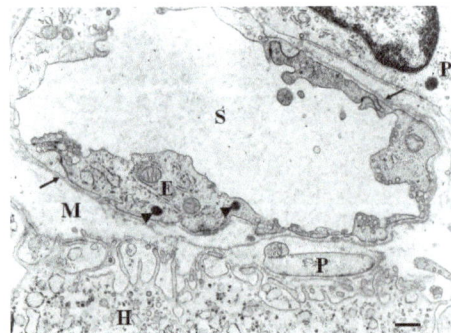

Fig. 3. A transmission electron micrograph showing a hepatic sinusoid in the human cirrhotic liver.
SECs show no fenestrae but contain many Weibel-Palade bodies (arrowheads) in the cytoplasm and continuous basement membranes (arrows) to the side. The Disse space is filled with the extracellular matrix. That is, typical hepatic sinusoidal capillarization is shown.
S: sinusoid, **E**: SEC, **P**: process of HSCs, **H**: hepatocyte, **M**: extracellular matrix

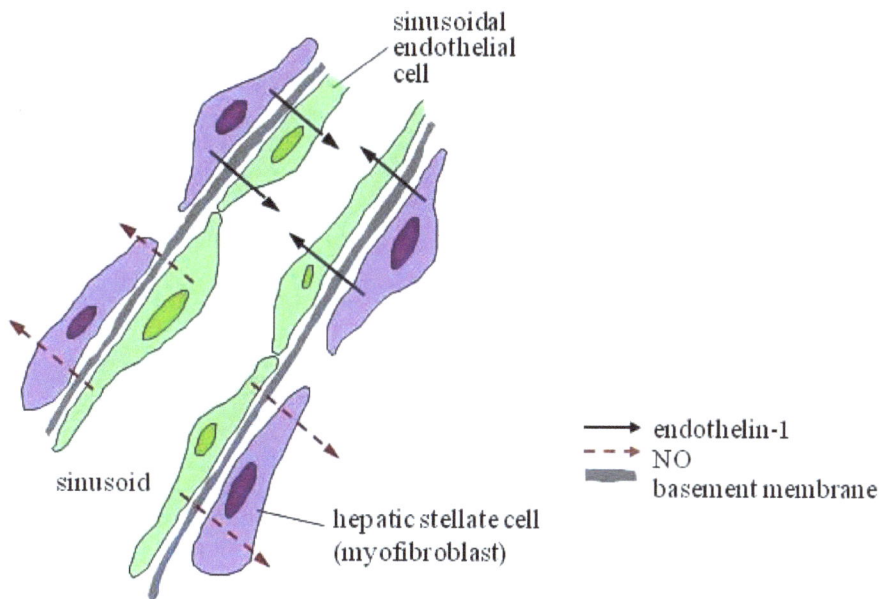

Fig. 4. A diagram showing the relationship between hepatic sinusoidal walls and vasoactive agents in the cirrhotic liver.

In the cirrhotic liver accompanied with the sinusoidal capillarization, the sinusoidal microcirculation is suggested to be primarily regulated by vasoactive agents such as ET-1 and NO in a paracrine and autocrine manner instead of neurotransmitters.

There are only a few reports on innervation of the cirrhotic liver. All publications conclude to a decreased density of nerves in the lobular space, as observed following immunolabeling for nerve markers [12, 23, 30]. On the other hand, it is also apparent that nerve fiber density is increased in fibrous portal tracts [23, 31] and also around portal veins in cases of alcoholic liver disease [30]. Matsunaga *et al.* [31] quantified the number of nerves/mm^2 stromal areas and found a more than 10-fold increase in severe chronic hepatitis B and C or autoimmune hepatitis and a 4-fold increase in alcoholic liver disease. The nature of this innervation has not been studied in detail. It is conceivable that these nerve endings are involved in the abnormal control of liver blood flow in chronic liver diseases. They could also modulate the phenotype activated fibrogenic cells in fibrous tracts through neurotransmitter release.

5. LIVER CIRRHOSIS-INDUCED PORTAL HYPERTENSION AND ESTROGEN

NO is produced in the liver by SECs, Kupffer cells, HSCs and hepatocytes. NO is produced by NOS, with L-arginine as the substrate. The cytoplasmic processes of HSCs in the Disse spaces surrounding the SECs. Portal hypertension is one of the main complications of liver cirrhosis (LC), and it is said to be caused by increased resistance in the blood vessels. The increased resistance in the blood vessels of the liver in LC is understood to be owing to a significant decrease in the production of NO in the liver along with a concomitant increase in endothelin-1, which is accompanied by the transformation of HSCs into myofibloblast-like cells.

On the other hand, it is known that serum estrogen levels are increased in patients with LC, and that this increased estrogen is closely related to palmer erythema, vascular spider and gynecomastia. Also, it has been reported that administration of 17β-estradiol inhibited the increase of HSCs and of collagen production, and improved liver fibrosis. Further, 17β-estradiol acting on vascular endothelial cells increased NOS activity, indicating the production of NO by vascular endothelial cells. We have previously reported that SECs also produce NO through the action of 17β-estradiol, similar to the vascular endothelial cells (Fig. **5**).

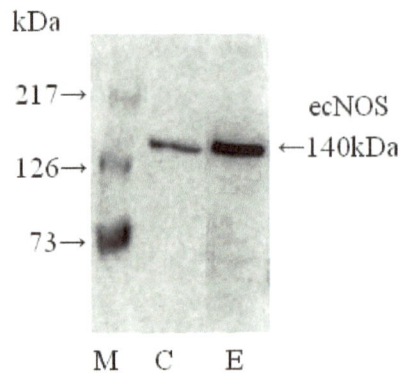

Fig. 5. Expression of ecNOS protein in the rat normal cultured SECs by Western blotting.
The ecNOS protein expression treated with 100 pg/mL 17β-estradiol for 24 h is increased compared with that in non-treated control HSCs.
M: medium, C: control, E: 17β-estradiol

That is, the effects of estrogen on Ca^{2+}/calmodulin-dependent endothelial cell NOS (eNOS) production were investigated using the cirrhosis model rats. Cirrhosis was induced by dimethylnitrosamine. Estradiol valerate was subcutaneously injected twice at week 4 after dimethylnitrosamine treatment. Furthermore, subcutaneous injection of an estrogen receptor antagonist, ICI-182780, was performed 2 days before administration of estradiol valerate. Portal pressure and hepatic blood flow were measured. NOS activity was assessed by l-citrulline generation. SECs were isolated from the cirrhotic rat livers and cultured. The cells were incubated with estradiol and /or ICI-182780 for 24 hours. Images for nitric oxide in SECs were obtained using diaminofluorescein-2 diacetate. In results, cirrhotic rats treated with estradiol valerate showed a significant decrease in portal pressure (Fig. **6**) and a significant increase in hepatic blood flow compared with those of control cirrhosis rats (Fig. **7**). However, in cirrhotic rats treated with ICI-182780, the reduction of portal pressure and elevation of hepatic blood flow were completely inhibited (Figs. **6** and **7**). In cirrhotic rats treated with estradiol valerate, NOS activity was increased compared with that in the control cirrhotic rats (Fig. **8**). The fluorescent level of intracellular NO in SECs stimulated by estradiol, and cultured was higher than that in non-treated SECs (Fig. **9**). From the results, estrogen plays an important role in the enhancement of nitric oxide production in SECs of cirrhotic liver and reduces the portal pressure in cirrhotic rats [32].

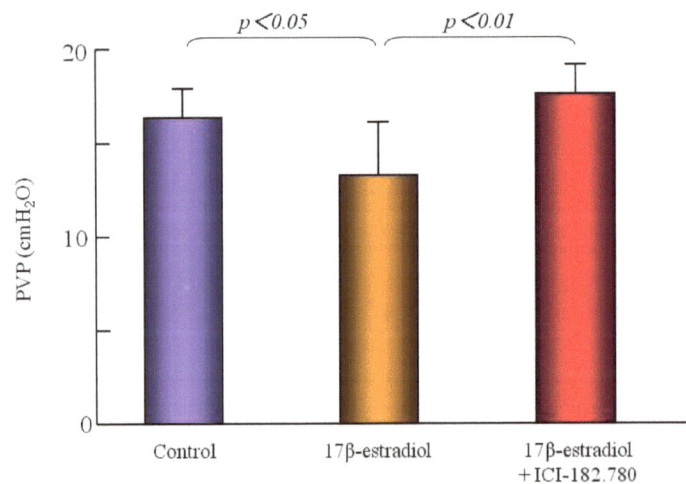

Fig. 6. Effect of 17β-estradiol on portal venous pressure (PVP) levels in dimethylnitrosamine-induced cirrhotic rats.
The PVP level is significantly lower in the 17β-estradiol treatment group (13.3 ± 1.8 cmH$_2$O) than in the control group (16.3 ± 1.6cmH$_2$O). However, the decrease in PVP level is significantly inhibited by ICI-182780 treatment (17.8 ± 1.7cmH$_2$O). Data are mean ± SD.

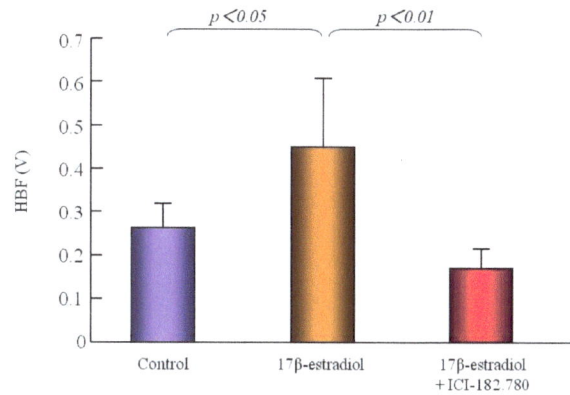

Fig. 7. Effect of 17β-estradiol on hepatic blood flow (HBF) levels in dimetylnitrosamine-induced cirrhotic rats. The HBF level is significantly higher in the 17β-estradiol treatment group (0.46 ± 0.16 V) than in the control group (0.27 ± 0.06 V). However, the increase in HBF level is significantly inhibited by ICI-182780 treatment (0.16 ± 0.05 V). Data are mean $\pm$ SD.

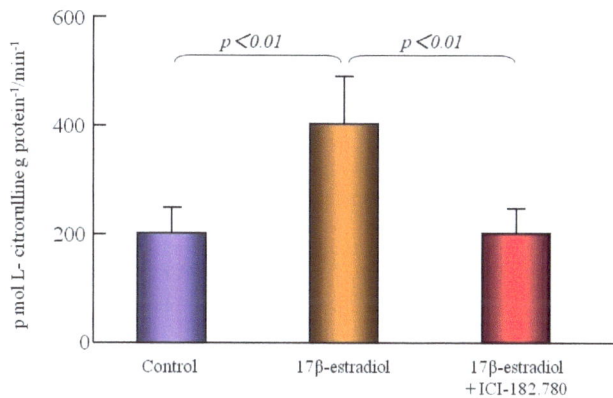

Fig. 8. Effect of 17β-estradiol on NOS levels in liver tissues of dimetylnitrosamine-induced cirrhotic rats. The NOS activity is significantly higher in the 17β-estradiol treatment group (380 ± 90) than in the control group (200 ± 40). However, the increase in NOS activity is significantly inhibited by ICI-182780 treatment (200 ± 50). Data are mean $\pm$ SD.

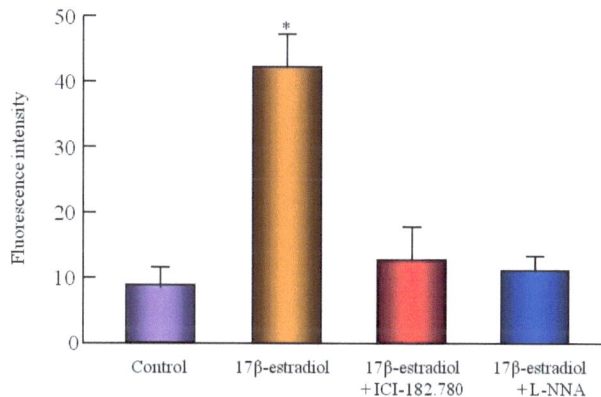

Fig. 9. Relative fluorescence intensity in cirrhotic cultured SECs 24 h after addition of 1 ng/mL 17β-estradiol to culture medium. The integrated DAF-2DA fluorescence intensity of the SECs is measured after treatment with 1 ng/mL 17β-estradiol, 1 ng/mL 17β-estradiol +1 μM ICI-182780, or 1 ng/mL 17β-estradiol + 100 μM NG-nitro-L-arginine (L-NMA). The fluorescence intensity is significantly higher in the 17β-estradiol treatment group (43 ± 4.5) than in the control group (9.4 ± 2.0). However, the effect is significantly inhibited by ICI-182780 (12.2 ± 2.9) or L-NMA treatment (10.9 ± 1.7). *$p < 0.001$ compared with the other groups. Data are mean $\pm$ SD.

In this study, there was no significant difference in eNOS protein expression in liver tissues between the 17β-estradiol-treated group and the non-treated group. This suggests the above-mentioned possibility that NOS activity was increased directly by estrogen, or that NOS activity was stimulated by non-genomic estrogen response. It is also reported that the administration of exogenous estrogen actually increases the number of ER, and may thereby promote the production of NO [33].

Men outnumber women among patients with liver cirrhosis by a ratio of 2.3 : 1. The higher production of cirrhosis among men is not necessarily related to the putative protective effects of estrogen but is mostly owing to the higher prevalence of certain etiologic factors in male patients, such as alcohol or chronic hepatitis C. it is also reported that the progression of hepatic fibrosis tends to occur sooner in men than in women [34-36]. Recent studies have reported that estrogen mediated by ERB inhibited the increase of HSCs and improved liver fibrosis [37], and that it is involved in increasing the sensitivity of Kupffer cells to endotoxin in pregnant women with severe hepatopathy [38].

6. CONCLUSION

Portal pressure is determined by extrahepatic factors such as portal blood flow and collateral resistance aside from intrahepatic resistance. The administration of 17β-estradiol lowered portal vein pressure and increased hepatic blood flow in cirrhotic model rats. It is considered that SECs in cirrhotic liver are stimulated by 17β-estradiol, and this was owing, at least in part, to the stimulation of NO produced by the SECs.

REFERENCES

[1]   Yanagisawa M, Kurihara H, Kimura S, *et al.* A novel potent vasoconstrictor peptide produced by vascular endothelial cells. Nature 1988; 332: 411-5.

[2]   Furchgott RF. Role of endothelium in responses of vascular smooth muscle. Circ Res 1983; 53: 557-73.

[3]   Huggins JP, Pelton JT, Miller RC. The structure and specificity of endothelin receptors: their importance in physiology and medicine. Pharmacol Ther 1993. 59: 55-123.

[4]   Eguchi S, Hirata Y, Imai T, Marumo F. Endothelin receptor subtypes are coupled to adenylate cyclase *via* different guanyl nucleotide-binding proteins in vasculature. Endocrinology 1993; 132: 524-9.

[5]   Tsukahara H, Ende H, Magazine HI, *et al.* Molecular and functional characterization of the non-isopeptide-selective ETB receptor in endothelial cells. Receptor coupling to nitric oxide synthase. J Biol Chem 1994; 269: 21778-85.

[6]   Douglas SA, Meek TD, Ohlstein EH. Novel receptor antagonists welcome a new era in endothelin biology. Trends Pharmacol Sci 1994; 15: 313-6.

[7]   Liu S, Premont RT, Kontos CD, *et al.* Endothelin-1 activates endothelial cell nitric-oxide synthase *via* heterotrimeric G-protein βγ subunit signaling to protein kinase B/Akt. J Biol Chem 2003; 278: 49929-35.

[8]   La Padula P, Bustamante J, Czerniczyniec A, Costa LE. Time course of regression of the protection conferred by simulated high altitude to rat myocardium: correlation with mtNOS. J Appl Physiol 2008; 105: 951-7.

[9]   Clemens MG, Zhang JX. Regulation of sinusoidal perfusion: *in vivo* methodology and control by endothelins. Semin Liver Dis 1999; 19: 383-96.

[10] Suematsu M, Wakabayashi Y, Ishimura Y. Gaseous monoxides: a new class of microvascular regulator in the liver. Cardiovasc Res 1996; 32: 679-86.

[11] Yokoyama Y, Nimura Y, Nagino M, *et al.* Current understanding of gender dimorphism in hepatic pathophysiology. J Surg Res 2005; 128: 147-56.

[12] Ueno T, Sata M, Sakata R, *et al.* Hepatic stellate cells and intralobular innervation in human liver cirrhosis. Hum Pathol 1997; 28:953-9.

[13] Geerts A. History, heterogeneity, developmental biology, and functions of quiescent hepatic stellate cells. Semin Liver Dis 2001; 21: 311-35.

[14] Ito T, Shibasaki S. Electron microscopic study on the hepatic sinusoidal wall and the fat-storing cells in the normal human liver. Arch Histol Jpn 1968; 29: 137-92.

[15] Ueno T, Inuzuka S, Torimura T, *et al.* Intrinsic innevation of the human liver. J Clin Electron Microscopy 1988; 21: 481-91.

[16]   Ueno T, Tanikawa K. Intralobular innervation and lipocyte contractility in the liver. Nutrition 1997; 13: 141-8.

[17]   Bioulac-Sage P, Lafon ME, Saric J, Balabaud C. Nerves and perisinusoidal cells in human liver. J Hepatol 1990; 10: 105-12.

[18]   Akiyoshi H, Gonda T, Terada T. A comparative histochemical and immunohistochemical study of aminergic, cholinergic and peptidergic innervation in rat, hamster, guinea pig, dog and human livers. Liver 1998; 18: 352-9.

[19]   Peinado MA, del Moral ML, Jiménez A, *et al.* The nitrergic autonomic innervation of the liver. Auton Neurosci 2002; 99: 67-9.

[20]   Moghimzadeh E, Nobin A, Rosengren E. Fluorescence microscopical and chemical characterization of the adrenergic innervation in mammalian liver tissue. Cell Tissue Res 1983; 230: 605-13.

[21]   Kyösola K, Penttila O, Ihamaki T, *et al.* Adrenergic innervation of the human liver. A fluorescence histochemical analysis of clinical liver biopsy specimens. Scand J Gastroenterol 1985; 20: 254-6.

[22]   Amenta F, Cavallotti C, Ferrante F, Tonelli F. Cholinergic nerves in the human liver. Histochem J 1981; 13: 419-24.

[23]   Miyazaki Y, Fukuda Y, Imoto M, *et al.* Immunohistochemical studies on the distribution of nerve fibers in chronic liver diseases. Am J Gastroenterol 1988; 83: 1108-14.

[24]   Lee JA, Ahmed Q, Hines JE, Burt AD. Disappearance of hepatic parenchymal nerves in human liver cirrhosis. Gut 1992; 33: 87-91.

[25]   El-Salhy M, Stenling R, Grimelius L. Peptidergic innervation and endocrine cells in the human liver. Scand J Gastroenterol 1993; 28: 809-15.

[26]   Sakamoto M, Ueno T, Kin M, *et al.* Ito cell contraction in response to endothelin-1 and substance P. Hepatology 1993; 18: 978-83.

[27]   Sakamoto M, Ueno T, Sugawara H, *et al.* Relaxing effect of interleukin-1 on rat cultured Ito cells. Hepatology 1997; 25: 1412-7.

[28]   Sakamoto M, Ueno T, Nakamura T, *et al.* Estrogen upregulates nitric oxide synthase expression in cultured rat hepatic sinusoidal endothelial cells. J Hepatol 2001; 34: 858-64.

[29]   Ueno T, Inuzuka S, Torimura T, *et al.* Serum hyaluronate reflects hepatic sinusoidal capillarization. Gastroenterology 1993; 105: 475-81.

[30]   Jaskiewicz K, Voigt MD, Robson SC. 1994. Distribution of hepatic nerve fibers in liver diseases. Digestion 1994 ; 55: 247-52.

[31]   Matsunaga Y, Kawasaki H, Terada T. Stromal mast cells and nerve fibers in various chronic liver diseases: relevance to hepatic fibrosis. Am J Gastroenterol 1999; 94: 1923-32.

[32]   Sakamoto M, Ueno T, Nakamura T, *et al.* Improvement of portal hypertension and hepatic blood flow in cirrhotic rats by oestrogen. Eur J Clin Invest 2005; 35: 220-5.

[33]   Shupnik MA, Gordon MS, Chin WW. Tissue-specific regulation of rat estrogen receptor mRNA. Mol Endocrinol 1989; 3: 660-5.

[34]   Yasuda M, Shimizu I, Shiba M, *et al.* Suppressive effects of estradiol on dimetylnitrosamine-induced fibrosis of the liver in rats. Hepatology 1999; 29: 719-27.

[35]   Zaman SN, Melia WM, Johnson RD, *et al.* Risk factors in development of hepatocellular carcinoma in cirrhosis: prospective study of 613 patients. Lancet 1985; 1: 1357-60.

[36]   Villa E, Baldini GM, Pasquinelli C, *et al.* Risk factors for hapatocellular carcinoma in Italy. Male sex, hepatitis B virus, non-A non-B infection, and alcohol. Cancer 1988; 62: 611-5.

[37]   Zhou Y, Shimizu I, Lu G, *et al.* Hepatic stellate cells contain the functional estrogen receptor beta but not the estrogen receptor alpha in male and female rats. Biochem Biophys Res Commun 2001; 286: 1059-65.

[38]   Ikejima K, Enomoto N, Iimuro Y, *et al.* Estrogen increases sensitivity of hepatic Kupffer cells to endotoxin. Am J Physiol 1998; 274: G669-76.

CHAPTER 9

Non-Alcoholic Fatty Liver Disease in Females and Males

Yosho Fukita, Tsutoshi Asaki, Yoshiki Katakura and Ichiro Shimizu[*]

Department of Gastroenterology, Seirei Yokohama Hospital, 215 Iwai-cho, Hodogaya-ku, Kanagawa 240-8521, Japan

Abstract: Increasing evidence indicates that hepatic fat accumulation is related to hepatic fibrosis, inflammation, apoptosis, and cancer. Males generally have larger visceral fat areas than females. Menopause is associated with a shift towards relatively more fat as well as towards the deposition of more fat in the abdominal region. Estrogen treatment of male-to-female transsexuals can increase the amount of subcutaneous adipose tissue; thus, estrogen changes the male type of visceral fat distribution into a female type of fat accumulation. Visceral fat accumulation arises through enlarged adipocytes, which release adiponectin, leptin, tumor necrosis factor-α (TNF-α), and fatty acids. Adiponectin inhibits the enlargement of adipocytes and fat accumulation. Adiponectin levels are consistently higher in females than in males. Persistent TNF-α stimuli lead to adipogenesis and impairment of mitochondria in hepatocytes and result in induction of oxidative stress. In experimental studies, when incubated with adiponectin, hepatic stellate cells undergo a number of antifibrogenic changes. Whereas leptin may play a role in the development of hepatic fibrosis. Hepatic steatosis spontaneously becomes evident in an aromatase-deficient mouse. Estrogen replacement reduces hepatic steatosis and restores the impairment in mitochondrial fatty acid β-oxidation to a wild-type level. In fact, tamoxifen, as an antiestrogen, has been shown to be associated with an increased risk of developing hepatic steatosis and non-alcoholic steatohepatitis (NASH) in non-obese female patients with breast cancer.

Understanding the sex-associated difference is necessary to inform the rational design of treatment strategies directed at visceral obese individuals who may develop from hepatic steatosis to cirrhosis and hepatocellular carcinoma.

Keywords: Non-alcoholic fatty liver disease, visceral fat accumulation, hepatic steatosis, NASH, TNF-α, estrogen, adiponectin, leptin, menopause, metabolic syndrome, BMI, obesity, fatty acid β-oxidation.

1. INTRODUCTION

Progression of hepatic fibrosis does not occur in a linear manner and several factors exert an influence, such as host factors of sex, age, duration of viral infection and consumption of alcohol. Currently, metabolic disorders such as being overweight and diabetes are emerging as cofactors of hepatic fibrosis. Fatty liver is considered the hepatic manifestation of the metabolic syndrome. The transition from premenopause to postmenopause is associated with the emergence of many features of the metabolic syndrome, including increased intra-abdominal (visceral) body fat, a shift towards a more atherogenic lipid profile and increased glucose and insulin levels. Visceral fat accumulation is a predictor of fatty liver. Furthermore, increasing evidence indicates that hepatic fat accumulation is related to hepatic fibrosis, inflammation, apoptosis, and cancer.

2. NON-ALCOHOLIC FATTY LIVER DISEASE IN FEMALES

Non-alcoholic fatty liver disease (NAFLD) is currently recognized as the most common form of chronic liver disease in many parts of the world. There is a growing concern regarding the development of NAFLD in clinical hepatology. Its name implies a histological picture that is indistinguishable from alcoholic liver disease. Fatty liver, which is also histologically called hepatic steatosis, is the result of the deposition of triglycerides *via* the accumulation of fatty acids in hepatocytes. Increased echogenicity ("bright" scan) with

*Address correspondence to Ichiro Shimizu: Department of Gastroenterology, Seirei Yokohama Hospital, 215 Iwai-cho, Hodogaya-ku, Yokohama, Kanagawa 240-8521, Japan; Tel: +81-45-715-3111; Fax: +81-45-715-3387; E-mail: ichiro.shimizu@showaclinic.jp

ultrasonography or increased radiolucency with computerized tomography (CT) compared with kidney provide supportive evidence of fatty liver [1] (Fig. **1**). Although in most cases, fatty liver does not progress to more severe liver diseases, approximately 15-20% of patients have histological signs of hepatic fibrosis and necroinflammation, indicating the presence of non-alcoholic steatohepatitis (NASH). In a "two hit" theory of NASH pathogenesis [2], the "first hit" of hepatic steatosis is followed by the "second hit" of oxidative stress and endotoxin (bacterial lipopolysaccharides)-induced proinflammatory stimuli, leading to cell death and progression to hepatic fibrosis and NASH. Hepatic fat accumulation leads to production of reactive oxygen species (ROS) caused by mitochondrial respiratory chain dysfunction and/or cytochrome P450 2E1 (CYP2E1) in the microsomes. CYP2E1 has a very high NADPH oxidase activity and extensively produces ROS. Endotoxins, one of the components of the outer wall of gram-negative bacteria in gastrointestinal tract, are detoxified in the reticuloendothelial system, particularly in macrophages and Kupffer cells in the liver. Kupffer cells stimulated by gut-derived endotoxin *via* the portal vein produce proinflammatory cytokines such as tumor necrosis factor-α (TNF-α). Patients with NASH are at higher risk for developing cirrhosis and its complications such as hepatocellular carcinoma (HCC) [3]. Therefore, NAFLD refers to a spectrum of histopathology, ranging from simple hepatic steatosis to NASH and the end-stage cirrhosis, all occurring in the absence of history of alcohol abuse defined as an alcohol intake of more than 20 g per day (Table **1**).

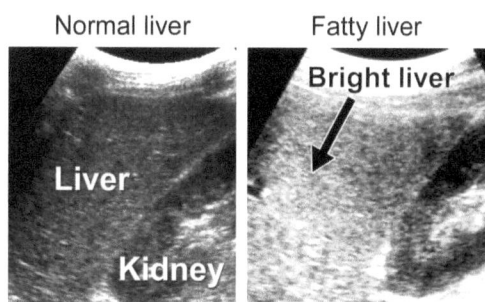

Fig. 1. Ultrasonographic findings of fatty liver. Fatty liver is detected by ultrasonography based on the comparative assessment of image brightness of the liver relative to the kidney.

Table 1. Spectrum of NAFLD

Simple hepatic steatosis	Excessive accumulation of triglycerides in hepatocytes, affecting at least 5% of the cells
NASH (non-alcoholic steatohepatitis)	Hepatic steatosis, cell death, hepatocyte ballooning, lobular inflammation, hepatic fibrosis
Cirrhosis	End-stage liver disease and its complications such as portal hypertension and hepatocellular carcinoma

Earlier impressions that NAFLD/NASH was a female-predominate condition have been dispelled; it actually appears to be more prevalent in males [4-6]. Data from the third National Health and Nutrition Survey (NHANES III) in the United States were estimated that 16% of adult females and 31% of adult males have NAFLD [5,7]. NAFLD has a very high prevalence in much of Europe, the Middle East (spanning southwestern Asia and northeastern Africa), Asia-Pacific (including Australia and New Zealand), and the United States. In most regions, ultrasonographic surveys of the general population indicate that almost one-quarter of the adult population has fatty liver [7,8]. NAFLD is more common in males than females, particularly in Asians [9]. In support of the sex difference in NAFLD among Asians, the incidence of ultrasonographic NAFLD was examined by sex and age in 3,229 Japanese adults from 2005 to 2006 in a health checkup center in Tokushima, western Japan (Fig. **2**). NAFLD was 2.5-fold more prevalent in males (31.5%) than in females (12.4%). Although NAFLD was more prevalent in females over the age of 70 years, the biggest difference in the prevalence of NAFLD between females and males was found in individuals of less than 50 years old [10]. Furthermore, among 3,175 Shanghai adults, the peak incidence of fatty liver in males occurred earlier (40-49 years) than in females (over 50 years) [11].

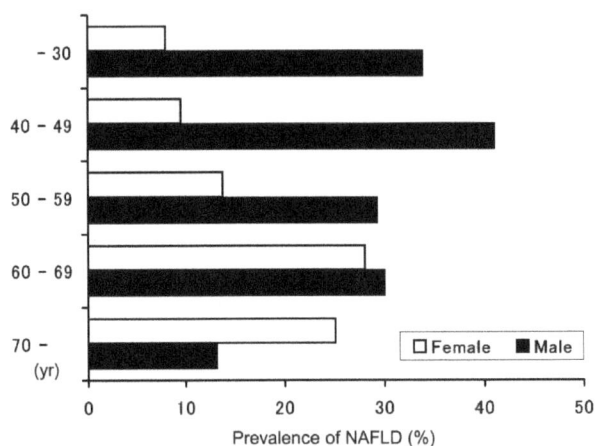

Fig. 2. Prevalence of NAFLD by gender and age. NAFLD prevalence was determined ultrasonogrraphically in 3,229 Japanese subjects (mean age 52.4 years, 45.9% males) in the Tokushima Health Checkup Center, in Japan. The subjects had no history of alcohol abuse, defined as an alcohol intake of more than 20 g per day, and were seronegative for hepatitis B surface antigen and the antibody to hepatitis C virus. The overall prevalence of NAFLD was 25.6%.

3. METABOLIC SYNDROME IN FEMALES

The prevalence of the metabolic syndrome increases with menopause and may partially explain the apparent acceleration in cardiovascular disease after menopause. In fact, coronary heart disease and stroke are rare before the menopause [12]. The transition from premenopause to postmenopause is associated with the emergence of many features of the metabolic syndrome, including increased visceral body fat, a shift towards a more atherogenic lipid profile and increased glucose and insulin levels (these conditions are known as peripheral insulin resistance). Obesity and diabetes, conditions associated with insulin resistance, are frequently observed in patients with NAFLD [13]. The incidence of increased visceral fat accumulation was quite low in females, particularly, aged less than 60 years old in a cohort study of local residents in Japan [14]. Increased fat accumulation areas ($\geq 100 cm^2$) were measured by CT. Visceral fat areas from a single CT scan obtained at the level of the umbilicus are correlated with the total visceral fat volume [15].

Based on data in 2002 from the National Nutrition Survey in Japan, increased blood levels of triglycerides (≥ 150 mg/dL) and hemoglobin A1c ($\geq 6.5\%$) and obese individuals (body mass index ≥ 25 kg/m^2) were more frequently observed in postmenopausal females and males (Fig. **3**). However, there was no significant difference of the incidences of abnormatily of hemoglobin A1c between female and male persons aged less than 50 yerars old. Hemoglobin A1c is used for screening and identification of impaired glucose tolerance and diabetes. A hemoglobin A1c of 6.5% shows the high sensitivity and specificity for diagnosing diabetes. Hemoglobin A1c and fasting blood glucose are found to be similarly effective in diagnosing diabetes.

However, obesity prevalence data in Japan indicate the tendency of females to be more obese than males, which is almost similar to those in other different parts of the world [16]. In Japanese females, the prevalence rate gradually increases to 30% in their 60s, and thereafter remains higher than in males. These differences are probably biologically based and relate to male's ability to deposit more lean (muscle) than fat tissue when energy imbalance occurs with weight gain. Females have more fat mass and less lean mass than males.

Table 2. Definitions of terms on BMI

Formula of BMI	BMI = body weight (in kg) ÷ height (in meters) squared
Normal weight	BMI $\geq$ 18.5 to 24.9 kg/m^2
Overweight	BMI $\geq$ 25.0 to 29.9 kg/m^2
Obesity	BMI $\geq$ 30 kg/m^2

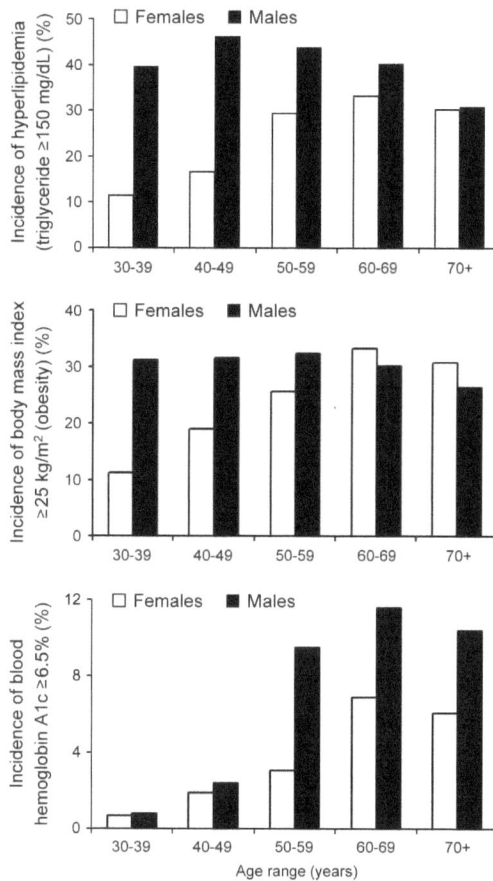

Fig. 3. Incidence of hypertriglyceridemia ($\geq$150 mg/dl) (upper panel), obese individuals (body mass index $\geq$ 25 kg/m^2) (middle panel), and increased blood hemoglobin A1c ($\geq$6.5%) (lower panel) based on data from the National Nutrition Survey in Japan.

Visceral fat accumulation, or visceral (central) obesity, is an independent predictor of hepatic steatosis, even in persons with a normal body mass index. Body mass index (BMI) is the most practical way to evaluate the overall degree of excess weight (Table **2**), which mainly reflects total body fat accumulation, or subcutaneous fat accumulation. Overweight and obesity are defined as BMI $\geq$ 25 to 29.9 kg/m^2 and $\geq$30 kg/m^2, respectively. Visceral fat accumulation is a more important factor for hepatic steatosis than BMI. It should be noted that regional fat distribution differs between females and males. After correction for total body fat mass, males generally have larger visceral fat areas than females [17] (Fig. **4**). Visceral fat accumulation (android pattern) is much more harmful than subcutaneous fat accumulation (gynoid pattern) [18,19]. Menopause is associated with a shift toward relatively more fat as well as toward the deposition of more fat in the abdominal region. In fact, starting within the first year from the menopause, females tend to gain weight and have a redistribution of body fat from a gynoid to an android pattern [20].

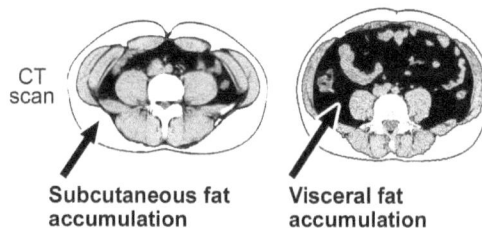

Fig. 4. Difference of regional fat distribution between females and males. Males generally have larger visceral fat areas than females. Visceral fat areas from a single CT scan obtained at the level of the umbilicus are correlated with the total visceral fat volume.

4. HEPATIC STEATOSIS AND OXIDATIVE STRESS

Increased lipid peroxidation and accumulation of end products of lipid peroxidation are commonly observed in NAFLD and alcoholic liver disease based on studies of human alcohol-related liver injury and animal models of diet-induced hepatic steatosis and drug-induced steatohepatitis [21-23]. Fatty liver is the result of the deposition of triglycerides *via* the accumulation of fatty acids in hepatocytes. In the progression of fatty liver disease, lipid peroxidation products are generated because of impaired β-oxidation of the accumulated fatty acids. The major site for fatty acid β-oxidation (degradation of fatty acids) in the liver is hepatocyte mitochondria (Fig. **5**). Key mediators of impaired fatty acid β-oxidation include a reduced mitochondrial electron transport (respiratory chain dysfunction). In addition to impaired mitochondrial β-oxidation of fatty acids, an activity of CYP2E1 in the microsomes is increased. Increased activity of CYP2E1 is found in the livers of obese animals [24] and NASH patients [4]. CYP2E1 catalyzes fatty acid ω-hydroxylations (microsomal ω-oxidation of fatty acids). Elevated CYP2E1 and mitochondrial defects result in an increase in the ROS formation and lipid peroxidation products. ROS and lipid peroxidation in turn cause further mitochondrial dysfunction and oxidative stress, thus contributing to cell death *via* ROS-induced DNA injury and membrane lipid peroxidation and discharge of products of lipid peroxidation, malondialdehyde (MDA) and 4-hydroxynonecal (HNE), into the space of Disse. MDA and HNE besides ROS are able to activate inflammatory cells (neutrophils, macrophages and Kupffer cells) and hepatic stellate cells (HSCs). Activated HSCs are responsible for much of the collagen synthesis observed during fibrosis development to the end-stage cirrhosis. Activated inflammatory cells in turn produce chemokines as well as TNF-α and ROS. Chemokines such as macrophage chemotactic protein-1 (MCP-1) and interleukin-8 (IL-8) attract neutrophils, lymphocytes, monocytes, macrophages, and Kupffer cells to inflammatory sites, leading to the persistent liver injury.

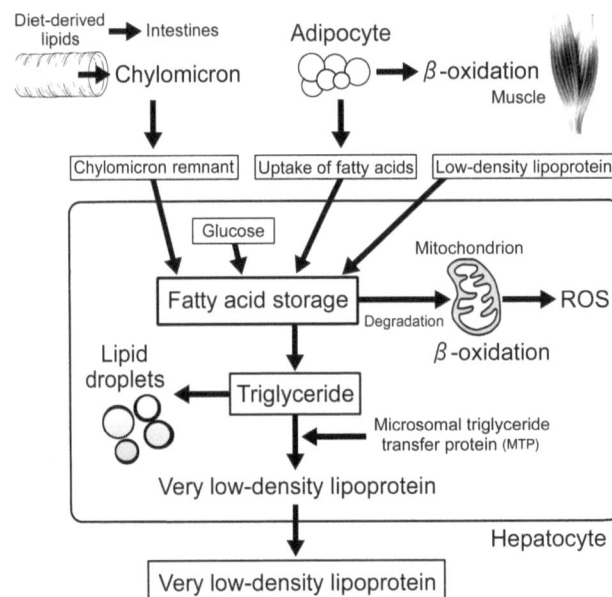

Fig. 5. Increased hepatic uptake of free fatty acids, increased triglyceride synthesis, and impaired transport of very low-density lipoprotein (triglyceride-rich lipoprotein) into the blood mainly contribute to the accumulation of hepatocellular triglycerides. Microsomal trigyceride transfer protein (MTP) is essential for the secretion of very low-density lipoprotein. Excess triglycerides are stored as lipid droplets in hepatocytes, which in turn results in a preferential shift to fatty acid degradation (β-oxidation), leading to the formation of ROS and lipid peroxidation products.

Mitochondrial defects may possibly have a genetic basis [25] and are likely worsened by aging and environmental factors such as high saturated fats [26,27]. Visceral fat accumulation arises through enlarged adipocytes. Adipocytes in visceral fat tissue release fatty acids and so called adipokines including adiponectin, leptin and TNF-α [28] (Table **3**). These adipokines and fatty acids flow directly into the liver *via* the portal vein, and they are involved in the development of metabolic syndrome and NAFLD. Mitochondrial dysfunction and oxidative stress are reported in the livers of patients with NASH [29]. Production of TNF-α and ROS by activated Kupffer cells and accumulated macrophages in the liver is also thought to play an important role in NASH-associated cirrhosis. Kupffer cells and macrophages are stimulated by gut-derived endotoxin *via* the portal vein, and produce a variety of cytokines such as TNF-α and interleukin-6 (IL-6). TNF-α is responsible, at least in part, for a number of pathophysiological responses in the liver, including ROS production, fat formation, insulin resistance, and hepatic fibrogenesis.

Table 3. Adipokines released by adipocytes

Adiponectin	Higher blood levels of adiponectin in females than in males; low blood levels of adiponectin in subjects with visceral fat accumulation; higher adiponectin levels in the olders than in the youngers; up-regulation of fatty acid β-oxidation and down-regulation of fatty acid production within hepatocytes; inhibition of activated HSC proliferation and fibrogenic function
Leptin	Higher blood levels of leptin in females than in males; strongest correlation with subcutaneous fat which secretes more leptin in comparison with visceral fat; no difference of leptin levels between premenopauses and postmenopauses
TNF-α	One of fat formation and insulin resistance inducible factors as well as proinflammatory cytokines

Cell injury may occur when the capacity of hepatocytes to safely store fat is overwhelmed by continued uptake [30], local synthesis, or impaired egress of fatty acids [31]; these fatty acids then become toxic to the cell in a pathobiological process termed lipotoxicity. Lipotoxicity can cause cell death by the direct effects of lipid mediators on apoptosis. Alternatively, liberation of oxidized lipids and their peroxidation products, such as chemotactic aldehydes and organic acids, may be instrumental in recruiting and perpetuating the inflammatory response that characterizes NASH. Fatty liver is predisposed to forms of injury that involve oxidative stress. Oxidative stress, TNF-α, other cytokines and chemokines are all present in NASH, but the ways in which they initiate or perpetuate steatohepatitis remain uncertain.

5. ADIPOKINES IN FEMALE

Adiponectin decreases in obese states, particularly with visceral obesity [32]. Blood adiponectin levels correlate inversely with visceral fat, fasting insulin concentrations and blood triglycerides [33]. Importantly, adiponectin levels are consistently higher in females than in males, independent of age and body fat [34]. These results are validated in adult populations inclusive of multiple ethnic groups such as Caucasians [34], Maoris [35], African Americans and Hispanics [36]. Adiponectin stimulates peroxisome proliferator-activated receptor α (PPARα) which has a number of beneficial effects including increased fatty acid β-oxidation, a reduction in hepatic triglycerides and inhibition of cytokines such as IL-6 [37]. Further anti-inflammatory effects of adiponectin are mediated *via* inhibition of macrophages and direct blockade of TNF-α release [38]. Such anti-steatotic and anti-inflammatory properties of adiponectin [39] may, in part, explain the decreased visceral fat accumulation and lower prevalence of fatty liver in females.

However, adiponectin levels in the older (> 51 years) group in a cohort in the United States were higher than in the younger (≤51 years) group, although the older individuals had greater visceral fat accumulation [34]. Two population studies demonstrated an inverse correlation between estrogen and adiponectin levels [40]. In addition, blood levels of total testosterone appear to correlate positively with blood adiponectin levels in both females and males, independent of measures of body fat [41]. Thus, estrogens alone are not responsible and may in fact have a negative rather than positive influence on circulating adiponectin levels.

Leptin plays a key role in the regulation of appetite and body weight. It also acts on the hypothalamus, altering energy intake by decreasing appetite and increasing energy expenditure *via* sympathetic stimulation of several tissues [39]. Blood leptin levels correlate well with body fat mass; this correlation is strongest for subcutaneous fat which secretes more leptin [42]. Although leptin levels are higher in premenopausal and postmenopausal females than in males even after adjustment for age and BMI [43], most studies show no difference of leptin levels between premenopausal and postmenopausal females when matched for BMI [44,45]. In contrast, testosterone inhibits leptin production by human adipocytes [44,46], and hypogonadal males (defined as the failure to produce androgens) have elevated leptin levels which are reduced by testosterone substitution [47]. These data suggest that sex differences in blood leptin levels appear to be due to an interaction between sex hormones and differences in body composition [37].

Increases in visceral adipose tissue and hepatic fat accumulation correlate with increased gluconeogenesis, increased free fatty acid levels, and insulin resistance [48]. Visceral fat accumulation is also associated with hepatic inflammation and fibrosis in patients with NASH independently of insulin resistance, an effect possibly mediated by IL-6 [49]. Increased expression of hepatic IL-6 correlated with insulin resistance in another report [50]. Several other adipokines such as TNF-α also involved in insulin receptor signaling appear to be altered in omental adipose tissue of NASH patients [51].

6. HEPATIC STEATOSIS IN CHRONIC HEPATITIS B AND C

Chronic hepatitis B and C are both frequently associated with hepatic steatosis. The frequency of hepatic steatosis in chronic hepatitis B ranges from 27 to 51%, while in chronic hepatitis C it is between 31 and 72% [52-55]. Hepatic steatosis is a characteristic feature of chronic hepatitis B virus (HBV) and hepatitis B virus (HCV) infections, suggesting that hepatic steatosis may reflect a direct cytopathic effect of hepatitis viruses and may play a role in the progression of the disease. In fact, a transgenic mouse model, which expressed the HCV core gene, develops progressive hepatic steatosis and HCC [56,57]. Chronic hepatitis C is commonly associated with hepatic steatosis [58], insulin resistance and diabetes [59]. A meta-analysis of over 3000 patients with hepatitis C shows that hepatic steatosis is a strong predictor of advanced disease [60]. It is conceivable that following hepatocyte injury, hepatic steatosis leads to an increase in lipid peroxidation, which may contribute to HSC activation by releasing soluble mediators [61] such as lipid peroxidation products, TNF-α and ROS, and thereby inducing hepatic fibrosis.

In contrast to HCV, there is little information on the correlation between HBV-associated hepatic steatosis and fibrosis. The molecular mechanism by which HBV mediates hepatic steatosis has not yet been clearly studied. Although a cross-sectional study in Australia failed to confirm the impact of hepatic steatosis on fibrosis in chronic hepatitis B, but not C [62], another cross-sectional analysis in Taiwanese adults revealed that HBV carrier status, ultrasonographic fatty liver and male sex are independently associated with liver damage evaluated by a conventional marker, blood alanine aminotransferase (ALT) level [63]. Moreover, hepatitis B x (HBx) protein induces hepatic fat accumulation mediated by sterol regulatory element binding protein 1 (SREBP-1) and peroxisome proliferator-activated receptor γ (PPARγ), leading to hepatic steatosis [64]. Increasing evidence indicates that hepatic fat accumulation is related to hepatic fibrosis, inflammation, apoptosis, and cancer [65,66].

In animal and *in vitro* studies, when incubated with adiponectin, HSCs undergo a number of antifibrogenic changes such as decreased the potent profibrogenic cytokine transforming growth factor-β (TGF-β) [67]. In obese leptin deficient mice, adiponectin treatment is associated with improvement in hepatic steatosis, liver enzyme levels and hepatic inflammation [68], while adiponectin knockout mice demonstrate enhanced hepatic fibrosis [67]. Currently, however, there is insufficient evidence to suggest that differential expression of adiponectin is enough to explain the better prognosis seen in females with chronic liver disease. Activated HSCs produce leptin [69], which is reported to up-regulate TNF-α, TGF-β and the expression of collagen type I [70]. Thus, leptin may play a role in the development of hepatic fibrosis. However, there is no evidence that the higher levels of leptin found in females may contribute to modulation of disease severity in NAFLD and chronic hepatitis B and C [71].

7. ESTRADIOL INHIBITS HEPATIC STEATOSIS

Fat accumulation is much more harmful in the visceral adipose tissue than in the subcutaneous adipose tissue [18,19]. Adipokines and fatty acids, derived from enlarged visceral adipcytes, flow directly into the liver *via* the portal vein, and they are involved in the development of metabolic syndrome and NAFLD.

Human adipose tissue contains estrogen receptor α and estrogen receptor β. Low estrogen levels in females with menopause are associated with a loss in subcutaneous fat and a gain in visceral fat [72]. In fact, starting within the first year from the menopause, females tend to have a redistribution of body fat from a gynoid to an android pattern. Estrogen treatment of male-to-female transsexuals can increase the amount of subcutaneous adipose tissue; thus, estrogen changes the male type of visceral fat distribution into a female type of fat accumulation [73]. Postmenopausal females treated with estrogen replacement are reported to have a lower visceral fat accumulation of adipose tissue in comparison to controls [74].

Patients with Turner's syndrome, which is characterized by estrogen deficiency, are associated with visceral obesity, increased liver enzyme ALT levels, and histologically proven NAFLD in up to 40% of cases [75-77]. Furthermore, a man with estrogen deficiency due to the aromatase gene inactivating mutation is reported to develop both steatohepatitis and insulin resistance, which are reversible with estradiol treatment [78]. Interestingly, polycystic ovary syndrome (PCOS) is associated with the development of NAFLD [79]. PCOS is a leading cause of infertility in premenopausal females. PCOS is a syndrome of ovarian dysfunction along with the cardinal features hyperandrogenism and polycystic ovary morphology. Its clinical manifestations may include menstrual irregularities, signs of androgen excess, and obesity [80,81]. In addition of the inhibitory role of estrogens in visceral fat accumulation and NAFLD development, androgen levels may also impact the NAFLD.

Microsomal triglyceride transfer protein (MTP) is essential and rate limiting for the assembly and secretion of very low-density lipoprotein (triglyceride-rich lipoprotein). Decreased hepatic expression of MTP contributes to the accumulation of hepatocellular triglycerides. Excess triglycerides are stored as lipid droplets in hepatocytes, leading to hepatic steatosis. Hepatic MTP expression is higher in females than in males, and this sex difference is regulated by the sexually dimorphic secretory pattern of growth hormone [82]. A continuous infusion of growth hormone increases MTP expression. Likely clinical manifestations of growth hormone deficiency in adults are increased visceral fat mass with a decrease in lean body mass. The profile of growth hormone secretion pattern also shows clear sex dimorphism [82]. In female rats, the growth hormone is continuously secreted, and the hormone levels are always detectable in the circulation, while, in male rats, it is secreted by episodic bursts every several hours with low or undetectable levels between peaks [83]. Integrated 24-hour growth hormone secretion [84] and fasting blood growth hormone levels (Fig. **6**) are higher in female individuals than in male individuals. Growth hormone secretion is stimulated by estrogens [82]. Oral and high-dose transdermal estrogen administration in menopausal females increases integrated 24-hour growth hormone secretion [85].

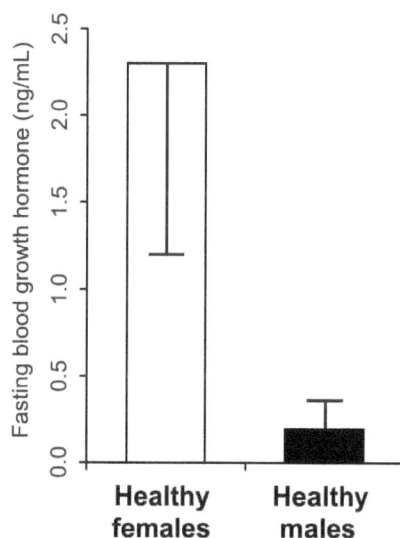

Fig. 6. Fasting mean blood levels of growth hormone in 15 premenopausal females (mean age 41.3 years) and 15 age-matched males (mean age 41.1 years) of healthy non-obese (BMI ≥ 18.5 to 24.9 kg/m^2) individuals. The subjects had no history of alcohol abuse (defined as an alcohol intake >20 g/day).

An experimental animal study showed that hepatic steatosis spontaneously becomes evident in an aromatase-deficient mouse, which lacks the intrinsic ability to produce estrogens and is impaired with respect to hepatic fatty acid β-oxidation. Estradiol replacement reduces hepatic steatosis and restores the impairment in mitochondrial and peroxisomal fatty acid β-oxidation to a wild-type level [86]. A preliminary study also demonstrated that estradiol stimulates gene expression of adiponectin in enlarged (matured) adipocytes [87]. Adiponectin inhibits the enlargement of visceral adipocytes and cellular fat accumulation. In primary cultures supplemented with lipids, estradiol inhibited TNF-α-induced fatty acid uptake into hepatocytes, and TNF-α-induced fat accumulation in hepatocytes was attenuated by estradiol.

Tamoxifen is a potent antagonist of estrogens, and it is used in the hormone treatment of estrogen receptor-positive breast cancer. Tamoxifen has been shown to be associated with an increased risk of developing hepatic steatosis and NASH in non-obese female patients with breast cancer [88,89]. In a clinical study from Japan, the frequency of tamoxifen-induced hepatic steatosis and NASH had increased to 36% [90]. These suggest that tamoxifen, as an antiestrogen, could suppress hepatic fatty acid β-oxidation and accelerate fat accumulation in hepatocytes. Therefore, the greater progression of liver injury with steatosis regardless of the etiology in males may be due, at least in part, to the decreased production of estradiol.

8. CONCLUSION

Over the last two decades, lifestyle changes have resulted in a dramatic increase in the prevalence of obesity in economically developed countries [91]. Organized physical activities, or purposeful exercise, such as walking, sport and physical play are now less popular than sedentary or 'spectator' activities, like television watching and internet surfing. More importantly, the minute-by-minute, hour-by-hour physical activities of everyday living (incidental activity) are dramatically reduced by modern lifestyle based on cars, household and building conveniences, and computer-based workstations [92]. Energy imbalance is responsible for excessive fat deposition. The increasing prevalence of obesity has also led to a higher incidence of metabolic syndrome including visceral obesity, hyperglycemia, hyperlipidemia and hypertension. The rising incidence of obesity and metabolic syndrome has occurred in paralleled with a dramatic increase of NAFLD.

Cirrhosis is 6 times more prevalent in obese individuals than in the general population [93]. Obesity, especially visceral obesity, is an independent risk factor in the development of NASH and HCC [94,95]. Visceral obesity is no longer a predictor of NAFLD/NASH, but rather is considered to be an essential risk factor for HCC. Higher risks associated with increased incidence and death rates for liver cancer are observed among obese males than among obese females [94,96]. Oxidative stress, proinflammatory cytokines, and other proinflammatory mediators as well as lipotoxicity may each play a role in transition of hepatic steatosis to NASH [97]. Patients with NASH who progress to cirrhosis are at increased risk of HCC. The second hit capable of inducing oxidative stress and proinflammatory stimuli in the first hit of hepatic steatosis is required for NASH, leading to cell death and progression to hepatic fibrosis and HCC [98].

It is important not only to diagnosis NASH in daily clinical practice but also to perform appropriate treatment taking into consideration the sex difference and influence of menopause in females. Understanding the sex-associated difference is necessary to inform the rational design of treatment strategies directed at visceral obese individuals who may develop from hepatic steatosis to cirrhosis and HCC.

REFERENCES

[1]   Saadeh S, Younossi ZM, Remer EM, *et al.* The utility of radiological imaging in nonalcoholic fatty liver disease. Gastroenterology 2002;123:745-50.

[2]   Brunt EM. Nonalcoholic steatohepatitis: definition and pathology. Semin Liver Dis 2001;21:3-16.

[3]   Harrison SA, Kadakia S, Lang KA, Schenker S. Nonalcoholic steatohepatitis: what we know in the new millennium. Am J Gastroenterol 2002;97:2714-24.

[4]   Weltman MD, Farrell GC, Hall P, *et al.* Hepatic cytochrome P450 2E1 is increased in patients with nonalcoholic steatohepatitis. Hepatology 1998;27:128-33.

[5] Clark JM, Brancati FL, Diehl AM. Nonalcoholic fatty liver disease. Gastroenterology 2002;122:1649-57.

[6] Browning JD, Szczepaniak LS, Dobbins R, *et al.* Prevalence of hepatic steatosis in an urban population in the United States: impact of ethnicity. Hepatology 2004;40:1387-95.

[7] Clark JM, Diehl AM. Defining nonalcoholic fatty liver disease: implications for epidemiologic studies. Gastroenterology 2003;124:248-50.

[8] Sanyal AJ. AGA technical review on nonalcoholic fatty liver disease. Gastroenterology 2002;123:1705-25.

[9] Weston SR, Leyden W, Murphy R, *et al.* Racial and ethnic distribution of nonalcoholic fatty liver in persons with newly diagnosed chronic liver disease. Hepatology 2005;41:372-9.

[10] Shimizu I, Kohno N, Tamaki K, *et al.* Female hepatology: favorable role of estrogen in chronic liver disease with hepatitis B virus infection. World J Gastroenterol 2007;13:4295-305.

[11] Fan JG, Zhu J, Li XJ, *et al.* Prevalence of and risk factors for fatty liver in a general population of Shanghai, China. J Hepatol 2005;43:508-14.

[12] Lerner DJ, Kannel WB. Patterns of coronary heart disease morbidity and mortality in the sexes: a 26-year follow-up of the Framingham population. Am Heart J 1986;111:383-90.

[13] Kim HJ, Kim HJ, Lee KE, *et al.* Metabolic significance of nonalcoholic fatty liver disease in nonobese, nondiabetic adults. Arch Intern Med 2004;164:2169-75.

[14] Koda M, Ando F, Niino N, Shimokata H. Relationship between age and visceral fat areas in a community-living population in Japan. J Geriatrics 2002;38:118.

[15] Sjostrom L, Kvist H, Cederblad A, Tylen U. Determination of total adipose tissue and body fat in women by computed tomography, 40K, and tritium. Am J Physiol 1986;250:E736-E745.

[16] James PT. Obesity: the worldwide epidemic. Clin Dermatol 2004;22:276-80.

[17] Elbers JM, Asscheman H, Seidell JC, Gooren LJ. Effects of sex steroid hormones on regional fat depots as assessed by magnetic resonance imaging in transsexuals. Am J Physiol 1999;276:E317-E325.

[18] Bellentani S, Saccoccio G, Masutti F, *et al.* Prevalence of and risk factors for hepatic steatosis in Northern Italy. Ann Intern Med 2000;132:112-7.

[19] Omagari K, Kadokawa Y, Masuda J, *et al.* Fatty liver in non-alcoholic non-overweight Japanese adults: incidence and clinical characteristics. J Gastroenterol Hepatol 2002;17:1098-105.

[20] Vitale C, Miceli M, Rosano GM. Gender-specific characteristics of atherosclerosis in menopausal women: risk factors, clinical course and strategies for prevention. Climacteric 2007;10 Suppl 2:16-20.

[21] Letteron P, Duchatelle V, Berson A, *et al.* Increased ethane exhalation, an *in vivo* index of lipid peroxidation, in alcohol-abusers. Gut 1993;34:409-14.

[22] Letteron P, Fromenty B, Terris B, *et al.* Acute and chronic hepatic steatosis lead to *in vivo* lipid peroxidation in mice. J Hepatol 1996;24:200-8.

[23] Berson A, De B, V, Letteron P, *et al.* Steatohepatitis-inducing drugs cause mitochondrial dysfunction and lipid peroxidation in rat hepatocytes. Gastroenterology 1998;114:764-74.

[24] Raucy JL, Lasker JM, Kraner JC, *et al.* Induction of cytochrome P450IIE1 in the obese overfed rat. Mol Pharmacol 1991;39:275-80.

[25] Petersen KF, Dufour S, Befroy D, *et al.* Impaired mitochondrial activity in the insulin-resistant offspring of patients with type 2 diabetes. N Engl J Med 2004;350:664-71.

[26] Petersen KF, Befroy D, Dufour S, *et al.* Mitochondrial dysfunction in the elderly: possible role in insulin resistance. Science 2003;300:1140-2.

[27] Lowell BB, Shulman GI. Mitochondrial dysfunction and type 2 diabetes. Science 2005;307:384-7.

[28] Czaja MJ. Liver injury in the setting of steatosis: crosstalk between adipokine and cytokine. Hepatology 2004;40:19-22.

[29] Sanyal AJ, Campbell-Sargent C, Mirshahi F, *et al.* Nonalcoholic steatohepatitis: association of insulin resistance and mitochondrial abnormalities. Gastroenterology 2001;120:1183-92.

[30] Donnelly KL, Smith CI, Schwarzenberg SJ, *et al.* Sources of fatty acids stored in liver and secreted *via* lipoproteins in patients with nonalcoholic fatty liver disease. J Clin Invest 2005;115:1343-51.

[31] Larter CZ, Farrell GC. Insulin resistance, adiponectin, cytokines in NASH: Which is the best target to treat? J Hepatol 2006;44:253-61.

[32] Whitehead JP, Richards AA, Hickman IJ, *et al.* Adiponectin--a key adipokine in the metabolic syndrome. Diabetes Obes Metab 2006;8:264-80.

[33] Lihn AS, Bruun JM, He G, *et al.* Lower expression of adiponectin mRNA in visceral adipose tissue in lean and obese subjects. Mol Cell Endocrinol 2004;219:9-15.

[34] Cnop M, Havel PJ, Utzschneider KM, *et al.* Relationship of adiponectin to body fat distribution, insulin sensitivity and plasma lipoproteins: evidence for independent roles of age and sex. Diabetologia 2003;46:459-69.

[35] Shand B, Elder P, Scott R, *et al.* Comparison of plasma adiponectin levels in New Zealand Maori and Caucasian individuals. N Z Med J 2007;120:U2606.

[36] Hanley AJ, Bowden D, Wagenknecht LE, *et al.* Associations of adiponectin with body fat distribution and insulin sensitivity in nondiabetic Hispanics and African-Americans. J Clin Endocrinol Metab 2007;92:2665-71.

[37] van der Poorten D, Milner KL, George J. Effect of adipokines on liver disease in females. In: Shimizu I, ed. Female Hepatology: Impact of female sex against progression of liver disease, Kerala, India: Research Signpost, 2009.

[38] Ouchi N, Kihara S, Arita Y, *et al.* Adiponectin, an adipocyte-derived plasma protein, inhibits endothelial NF-kappaB signaling through a cAMP-dependent pathway. Circulation 2000;102:1296-301.

[39] Kamada Y, Takehara T, Hayashi N. Adipocytokines and liver disease. J Gastroenterol 2008;43:811-22.

[40] Im JA, Lee JW, Lee HR, Lee DC. Plasma adiponectin levels in postmenopausal women with or without long-term hormone therapy. Maturitas 2006;54:65-71.

[41] Isobe T, Saitoh S, Takagi S, *et al.* Influence of gender, age and renal function on plasma adiponectin level: the Tanno and Sobetsu study. Eur J Endocrinol 2005;153:91-8.

[42] Van H, V, Reynisdottir S, Eriksson P, *et al.* Leptin secretion from subcutaneous and visceral adipose tissue in women. Diabetes 1998;47:913-7.

[43] Havel PJ, Kasim-Karakas S, Dubuc GR, *et al.* Gender differences in plasma leptin concentrations. Nat Med 1996;2:949-50.

[44] Haffner SM, Mykkanen L, Stern MP. Leptin concentrations in women in the San Antonio Heart Study: effect of menopausal status and postmenopausal hormone replacement therapy. Am J Epidemiol 1997;146:581-5.

[45] Bennett PA, Lindell K, Karlsson C, *et al.* Differential expression and regulation of leptin receptor isoforms in the rat brain: effects of fasting and oestrogen. Neuroendocrinology 1998;67:29-36.

[46] Wabitsch M, Blum WF, Muche R, *et al.* Contribution of androgens to the gender difference in leptin production in obese children and adolescents. J Clin Invest 1997;100:808-13.

[47] Jockenhovel F, Blum WF, Vogel E, *et al.* Testosterone substitution normalizes elevated serum leptin levels in hypogonadal men. J Clin Endocrinol Metab 1997;82:2510-3.

[48] Gastaldelli A, Cusi K, Pettiti M, *et al.* Relationship between hepatic/visceral fat and hepatic insulin resistance in nondiabetic and type 2 diabetic subjects. Gastroenterology 2007;133:496-506.

[49] van der PD, Milner KL, Hui J, *et al.* Visceral fat: a key mediator of steatohepatitis in metabolic liver disease. Hepatology 2008;48:449-57.

[50] Wieckowska A, Papouchado BG, Li Z, *et al.* Increased hepatic and circulating interleukin-6 levels in human nonalcoholic steatohepatitis. Am J Gastroenterol 2008;103:1372-9.

[51] Calvert VS, Collantes R, Elariny H, *et al.* A systems biology approach to the pathogenesis of obesity-related nonalcoholic fatty liver disease using reverse phase protein microarrays for multiplexed cell signaling analysis. Hepatology 2007;46:166-72.

[52] Scheuer PJ, Ashrafzadeh P, Sherlock S, *et al.* The pathology of hepatitis C. Hepatology 1992;15:567-71.

[53] Bach N, Thung SN, Schaffner F. The histological features of chronic hepatitis C and autoimmune chronic hepatitis: a comparative analysis. Hepatology 1992;15:572-7.

[54] Lefkowitch JH, Schiff ER, Davis GL, *et al.* Pathological diagnosis of chronic hepatitis C: a multicenter comparative study with chronic hepatitis B. The Hepatitis Interventional Therapy Group. Gastroenterology 1993;104:595-603.

[55] Czaja AJ, Carpenter HA. Sensitivity, specificity, and predictability of biopsy interpretations in chronic hepatitis. Gastroenterology 1993;105:1824-32.

[56] Moriya K, Yotsuyanagi H, Shintani Y, *et al.* Hepatitis C virus core protein induces hepatic steatosis in transgenic mice. J Gen Virol 1997;78 (Pt 7):1527-31.

[57] Moriya K, Fujie H, Shintani Y, *et al.* The core protein of hepatitis C virus induces hepatocellular carcinoma in transgenic mice. Nat Med 1998;4:1065-7.

[58] Asselah T, Rubbia-Brandt L, Marcellin P, Negro F. Steatosis in chronic hepatitis C: why does it really matter? Gut 2006;55:123-30.

[59] Shintani Y, Fujie H, Miyoshi H, *et al.* Hepatitis C virus infection and diabetes: direct involvement of the virus in the development of insulin resistance. Gastroenterology 2004;126:840-8.

[60]   Leandro G, Mangia A, Hui J, *et al.* Relationship between steatosis, inflammation, and fibrosis in chronic hepatitis C: a meta-analysis of individual patient data. Gastroenterology 2006;130:1636-42.

[61]   Gressner AM, Lotfi S, Gressner G, Lahme B. Identification and partial characterization of a hepatocyte-derived factor promoting proliferation of cultured fat-storing cells (parasinusoidal lipocytes). Hepatology 1992;16:1250-66.

[62]   Gordon A, McLean CA, Pedersen JS, *et al.* Hepatic steatosis in chronic hepatitis B and C: predictors, distribution and effect on fibrosis. J Hepatol 2005;43:38-44.

[63]   Lin YC, Hsiao ST, Chen JD. Sonographic fatty liver and hepatitis B virus carrier status: synergistic effect on liver damage in Taiwanese adults. World J Gastroenterol 2007;13:1805-10.

[64]   Kim KH, Shin HJ, Kim K, *et al.* Hepatitis B virus X protein induces hepatic steatosis *via* transcriptional activation of SREBP1 and PPARgamma. Gastroenterology 2007;132:1955-67.

[65]   Ohata K, Hamasaki K, Toriyama K, *et al.* Hepatic steatosis is a risk factor for hepatocellular carcinoma in patients with chronic hepatitis C virus infection. Cancer 2003;97:3036-43.

[66]   Powell EE, Jonsson JR, Clouston AD. Steatosis: co-factor in other liver diseases. Hepatology 2005;42:5-13.

[67]   Kamada Y, Tamura S, Kiso S, *et al.* Enhanced carbon tetrachloride-induced liver fibrosis in mice lacking adiponectin. Gastroenterology 2003;125:1796-807.

[68]   Xu A, Wang Y, Keshaw H, *et al.* The fat-derived hormone adiponectin alleviates alcoholic and nonalcoholic fatty liver diseases in mice. J Clin Invest 2003;112:91-100.

[69]   Potter JJ, Womack L, Mezey E, Anania FA. Transdifferentiation of rat hepatic stellate cells results in leptin expression. Biochem Biophys Res Commun 1998;244:178-82.

[70]   Aleffi S, Petrai I, Bertolani C, *et al.* Upregulation of proinflammatory and proangiogenic cytokines by leptin in human hepatic stellate cells. Hepatology 2005;42:1339-48.

[71]   van der Poorten D, Milner KL, George J. Effect of adipokines on liver disease in females. In: Shimizu I, ed. Female Hepatology: Impact of female sex against progression of liver disease, Kerala, India: Research Signpost, 2009.

[72]   Toth MJ, Tchernof A, Sites CK, Poehlman ET. Effect of menopausal status on body composition and abdominal fat distribution. Int J Obes Relat Metab Disord 2000;24:226-31.

[73]   Elbers JM, Asscheman H, Seidell JC, Gooren LJ. Effects of sex steroid hormones on regional fat depots as assessed by magnetic resonance imaging in transsexuals. Am J Physiol 1999;276:E317-E325.

[74]   Haarbo J, Marslew U, Gotfredsen A, Christiansen C. Postmenopausal hormone replacement therapy prevents central distribution of body fat after menopause. Metabolism 1991;40:1323-6.

[75]   Roulot D, Degott C, Chazouilleres O, *et al.* Vascular involvement of the liver in Turner's syndrome. Hepatology 2004;39:239-47.

[76]   Ostberg JE, Thomas EL, Hamilton G, *et al.* Excess visceral and hepatic adipose tissue in Turner syndrome determined by magnetic resonance imaging: estrogen deficiency associated with hepatic adipose content. J Clin Endocrinol Metab 2005;90:2631-5.

[77]   Lonardo A, Carani C, Carulli N, Loria P. 'Endocrine NAFLD' a hormonocentric perspective of nonalcoholic fatty liver disease pathogenesis. J Hepatol 2006;44:1196-207.

[78]   Maffei L, Murata Y, Rochira V, *et al.* Dysmetabolic syndrome in a man with a novel mutation of the aromatase gene: effects of testosterone, alendronate, and estradiol treatment. J Clin Endocrinol Metab 2004;89:61-70.

[79]   Cerda C, Perez-Ayuso RM, Riquelme A, *et al.* Nonalcoholic fatty liver disease in women with polycystic ovary syndrome. J Hepatol 2007;47:412-7.

[80]   Revised 2003 consensus on diagnostic criteria and long-term health risks related to polycystic ovary syndrome. Fertil Steril 2004;81:19-25.

[81]   Azziz R, Carmina E, Dewailly D, *et al.* Positions statement: criteria for defining polycystic ovary syndrome as a predominantly hyperandrogenic syndrome: an Androgen Excess Society guideline. J Clin Endocrinol Metab 2006;91:4237-45.

[82]   Ameen C, Oscarsson J. Sex difference in hepatic microsomal triglyceride transfer protein expression is determined by the growth hormone secretory pattern in the rat. Endocrinology 2003;144:3914-21.

[83]   Shapiro BH, Agrawal AK, Pampori NA. Gender differences in drug metabolism regulated by growth hormone. Int J Biochem Cell Biol 1995;27:9-20.

[84]   Clasey JL, Weltman A, Patrie J, *et al.* Abdominal visceral fat and fasting insulin are important predictors of 24-hour GH release independent of age, gender, and other physiological factors. J Clin Endocrinol Metab 2001;86:3845-52.

[85]   Friend KE, Hartman ML, Pezzoli SS, *et al.* Both oral and transdermal estrogen increase growth hormone release in postmenopausal women--a clinical research center study. J Clin Endocrinol Metab 1996;81:2250-6.

[86]   Nemoto Y, Toda K, Ono M, *et al.* Altered expression of fatty acid-metabolizing enzymes in aromatase- deficient mice. J Clin Invest 2000;105:1819-25.

[87]   Takenaka H, Shimizu I, Huang H, *et al.* Impact of estradiol on the sex-associated difference of fatty liver. Gastroenterology 2007;132:A-819.

[88]   Van HM, Rahier J, Horsmans Y. Tamoxifen-induced steatohepatitis. Ann Intern Med 1996;124:855-6.

[89]   Oien KA, Moffat D, Curry GW, *et al.* Cirrhosis with steatohepatitis after adjuvant tamoxifen. Lancet 1999;353:36-7.

[90]   Saibara T, Onishi S, Ogawa Y, *et al.* Non-alcoholic steatohepatitis. Lancet 1999;354:1299-300.

[91]   Zimmet P, Alberti KG, Shaw J. Global and societal implications of the diabetes epidemic. Nature 2001;414:782-7.

[92]   Farrell GC. Hepatitis C, other liver disorders, and liver health: a practical guide. Sydney: MacLennan & Petty Pty, 2002.

[93]   Ratziu V, Giral P, Charlotte F, *et al.* Liver fibrosis in overweight patients. Gastroenterology 2000;118:1117-23.

[94]   Calle EE, Rodriguez C, Walker-Thurmond K, Thun MJ. Overweight, obesity, and mortality from cancer in a prospectively studied cohort of U.S. adults. N Engl J Med 2003;348:1625-38.

[95]   Yalniz M, Bahcecioglu IH, Ataseven H, *et al.* Serum adipokine and ghrelin levels in nonalcoholic steatohepatitis. Mediators Inflamm 2006;2006:34295.

[96]   Wolk A, Gridley G, Svensson M, *et al.* A prospective study of obesity and cancer risk (Sweden). Cancer Causes Control 2001;12:13-21.

[97]   Farrell GC, Larter CZ. Nonalcoholic fatty liver disease: from steatosis to cirrhosis. Hepatology 2006;43:S99-S112.

[98]   Bugianesi E, Leone N, Vanni E, *et al.* Expanding the natural history of nonalcoholic steatohepatitis: from cryptogenic cirrhosis to hepatocellular carcinoma. Gastroenterology 2002;123:134-40.

CHAPTER 10

Sex and Gender Specific Medicine in Chronic Liver Diseases

Sumiko Nagoshi*

Department of Gastroenterology & Hepatology, Saitama Medical University, 38 Morohongo, Moroyama-machi, Iruma-gun, Saitama, 350-0495, Japan

Abstract: Sex and gender specific medicine is one of the most important issues to be promoted in recent medical care, from the viewpoint of the establishment of evidence-based medicine for the best therapies as well as patients' quality of life and also national health economics. Medical doctors should understand and elucidate the mechanisms underlying sex or gender differences regarding the incidence or etiology, clinical features, and each natural history or response to specific therapies.

Sex or gender differences have been generally observed among various liver diseases, such as viral hepatitis, alcoholic liver disease, non-alcoholic fatty liver disease, autoimmune hepatitis, primary biliary cirrhosis, primary sclerosing cholangitis and hepatocellular carcinoma. The mechanisms of these differences, however, are still obscure in spite of the world-wide reports, probably because there are variances in the regions, suggesting that such differences seem to exist in racial genes and cultural life style.

In this chapter, sex and gender specific medicine in the category of chronic liver diseases is reviewed by going through related original papers with personal opinions and comments.

Keywords: Hepatitis B virus, hepatitis C virus, viral hepatitis, alcoholic liver disease, non-alcoholic fatty liver disease, non-alcoholic steatohepatitis, autoimmune hepatitis, primary biliary cirrhosis, primary sclerosing cholangitis, hepatocellular carcinoma, cytochrome P4502E1, IL-6.

1. INTRODUCTION

The importance of sex and gender specific medicine in medical care has been recognized in recent years, and a number of studies related to the sex or gender differences have been piled up in the etiology, diagnosis, therapy, and prophylaxis of various diseases, and taken up as special reviews in the fields of cardiac disease, diabetes, hyperlipidemia, autoimmune disease, osteoporosis, pharmacokinetics, pharmacodynamics, and psychiatric disease, whereas sex and gender differences in human diseases frequently take on various aspects depending on the group cultures, geographic variances of humans or pathogens. Therefore, sex and gender specific medicine is an up-to-date medical issue to be established from the standpoint of bio-sociology and bio-economics, including racial and geographic cultures.

The International Society of Gender Medicine (IGM) was founded in 2006 as international, multidisciplinary, scientific organization with the purpose to develop sex and gender specific medicine in an international context by promoting gender aspects in science, research and public health. IGM has organized the annual meeting of International Congress on Gender Medicine. Also in Japan, the Japanese Association for Gender Specific Medicine was organized in 2004. In these past meetings, there were few reports regarding sex and gender specific medicine in liver diseases despite of its progress. Hepatologists are obliged not only to promote sex and gender specific medicine in hepatology, but also to propagate its basic and clinical information to the medical and general public.

2. VIRAL HEPATITIS

The prevalence of hepatitis B surface antigen (HBsAg) was reported to be higher in men as compared with women throughout the world [1]. An analysis of 3,485,648 first-time blood donors in Japan showed

*Address correspondence to Sumiko Nagoshi: Department of Gastroenterology & Hepatology, Saitama Medical University, 38 Morohongo, Moroyama-machi, Iruma-gun, Saitama, 350-0495, Japan; Tel: +81-49-276-1198; Fax: +81-49-276-1198; E-mail: snagoshi@saitama-med.ac.jp

Ichiro Shimizu (Ed)

positive HBsAg in blood to be significantly more frequent in male donors (0.73%) than in female donors (0.53%), while the antibody to hepatitis C virus (anti-HCV) was equally detected in men (0.48%) and women (0.50%) [2]. Considering that the main route of chronic infection with hepatitis B virus (HBV) in Japan is vertical transmission, which seems to occur equally between sexes, HBV is more likely to be eliminated in women than in men. It was also reported that having HBsAg was significantly more prevalent in men (9.7%) than in women (5.4%) in Okinawa [3]. In the follow-up study of up to 19 years (mean =9.2 years) in 946 HBsAg carriers in Okinawa, clearance of HBsAg was seen more frequently in women (7.8%) than in men (5.8%) [4]. Females have higher immunoglobulin levels than males, and estrogen treatment induced polyclonal B cell activation *in vitro* [5]. These effects might contribute to higher ability of females in eliminating HBsAg.

An analysis of 342,407 apparently healthy blood donors in Japan showed that positive hepatitis B e-antigen (HBeAg) was significantly more frequent in male donors (19.1%) as compared with female donors (16.7%), and that the rate of having the antibody to HBeAg was significantly less in men (49.6%) than in women (53.1%) among 6,342 asymptomatic HBV carriers [6]. In contrast, a study with 3,063 Chinese patients who had chronic hepatitis B infection showed no sex or gender difference in the spontaneous seroconversion rate of HBeAg to its antibody [7].

It was reported that HBeAg was signifinantly less prevalent in patients infected with HBV genotype B than in those infected with genotype C or A in Japan [8]. Furthermore, the annual seroconversion rate was significantly lower in children with vertical transmission compared with horizontal transmission in Greece [9]. These may explain the variance in the regions regarding sex or gender differences.

Multivariate analyses in the prospective study demonstrated that male sex and genotype C were significant predictive factors for reactivation of hepatitis B following HBeAg seroconversion in Taiwan [10]. The rate of progression to liver cirrhosis in 105 HBsAg-positive patients for 1-16 years was 24% in men and 8% in women [11]. These data suggest that female patients are more likely to undergo clinical remission and slow progression compared with males.

It is known that 60- 80% of adults infected with HCV progress to chronic hepatitis. In addition, the rate of HCV clearance was significantly higher in women (44.6%) than in men (33.7%), based on the data of 4,720 residents in Egypt, in which "cleared HCV" was defined as the case showing as positive in the anti-HCV antibody and no sign of HCV RNA in blood [12]. A study conducted in five European countries showed that sex was identified as one of the risk factors for HCV transmission to health care workers after exposure to blood or infectious body fluids from anti-HCV antibody-positive sources through percutaneous injuries (odds ratio for males *vs* females, 3.1) [13].

In chronic hepatitis C infection, the serum alanine aminotransferase (ALT) level was reported to be significantly higher in men than in women, only when the inflammatory activity was mild (A0-A1), and was significantly higher in younger patients than in older patients when the activity was more severe (A2-A3) [14]. We also reported that there were sex or gender differences in serum ALT levels between the low and high groups (Fig. **1**) [15]. Multivariate logistic regression analysis revealed that the important factor affecting hepatits activity was female sex [15]. Moreover, the progression time from HCV infection to liver cirrhosis was longer in women than in men [16-19], whereas no sex or gender differences were seen in some reports [20-22].

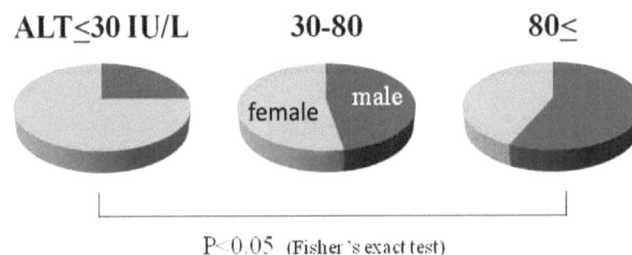

Fig. 1. Sex or gender difference in serum ALT level in chronic hepatitis C patients (modified from ref. 15)

The sustained virological response (SVR) rate to combination therapy with pegylated interferon α2b and ribavirin for 48 weeks showed no sex differences in patients with HCV genotype 1b under 50 years of age, although the SVR rate was significantly higher in men (51%) than in women (20%) in those aged over 50 years in Japan [23]. In contrast, in US patients between the ages of 18 and 70 years given such combination therapy, the SVR rate was significantly higher in women than in men [24]. This discrepancy may be due to the differences in the age of patients and the extent of hepatic fibrosis. Genetic factors in patients or HBV may be also related to the discrepancy. Recently, Tanaka Y *et al.* found that SNPs near the gene IL28B are strongly associated with null virological response (NVR) for such combination therapy in Japanese patients with HCV genotype 1b [25]. Indeed, there were ethnic differences in the frequency of the IL28B SNP alleles leading to NVR [26]. However, female sex and the allele were independent factors associated with NVR by logistic regression model [25].

3. ALCOHOLIC LIVER DISEASE

The incidence of alcoholic liver disease increases in a dose-dependent manner proportionally to the cumulative alcohol intake. Becker *et al.* reported that alcohol-induced liver disease developed more rapidly in women than in men [27]. The lowest point of daily alcohol intake for the development of liver disease was higher in men (24-48 g) than in women (12-24 g). In case of heavy drinkers with a daily consumption of 48-70 g, the relative risk of developing liver cirrhosis was 7 in men and 17 in women, and the relative risk for alcoholic liver disease was 3.7 in men and 7.3 in women. The factors affecting the differences in susceptibility to alcoholic toxicity, the age at the time of the regular consumption of alcohol, the way of drinking (that is, with or without meals), or the nutritional status may differently affect men and women.

There are several explanations for the mechanisms behind sex or gender differences in alcoholic liver disease. If one consumes the same amount of alcohol per body weight, the blood ethanol concentration would be higher in women than in men [28]. It was also reported that alcohol dehydrogenase (ADH), an enzyme involved in alcohol metabolism, was expressed at lower levels in the stomach in women as compared with men, and that the activity of gastric ADH was correlated with the gastric first-pass ethanol metabolism, affecting the blood ethanol concentration [28]. Baraona *et al.* stated that the sex or gender difference in the first-pass metabolism of ethanol was mainly due to lower gastric ADH activity in women than in men [29].

Thurman RG *et al.* reported that levels of plasma endotoxin, free radical adducts and infiltrating neutrophils in the liver were doubled in female rats compared with male rats after ethanol treatment [30]. Moreover, estrogen treatment *in vivo* increased the sensitivity of hepatic macrophages or Kupffer cells to endotoxin. They also presented the hypothesis that ethanol-induced liver injury involves elevations in circulating endotoxin levels leading to activation of Kupffer cells, which causes a hypoxia-reoxygenation injury [30]. These data suggested that Kupffer cells contribute to the sex or gender differences in alcoholic liver injury.

The administration of ethanol increased the hepatic activity of cytochrome P4502E1 (CYP2E1), known to be related to alcohol-induced oxidative stress, in female rats, and the ethanol-induced CYP2E1 activity was significantly reduced after the administration of anti-estrogen [31]. Ethanol feeding also increased the immuno-detectable CYP2E1 more abundantly in castrated micropigs than in non-castrated micropigs [32]. In addition, there was a significant correlation between the hepatic CYP2E1 level and serum 17-β-estradiol level in castrated micropigs after feeding ethanol [32].

4. NON-ALCOHOLIC FATTY LIVER DISEASE

The prevalence of non-alcoholic fatty liver disease (NAFLD) has been shown to be higher in men than in women in Asia [33]. However, some studies indicate an age-related trend. The prevalence of fatty liver was 25-30% in all of the age groups between 30 and 60 years in men, while the prevalence was 10% or less in the 30-39-year age group and increased gradually with age in 39,151 women who visited the Japanese health check-up center [34]. In women over the age of 70 years, fatty liver was more prevalent. A high body mass index was assumed to be one feature closely related to the onset of fatty liver, while alcohol intake did not show any clear relation to fatty liver [34]. Among 3,175 Shanghai adults, the peak prevalence of fatty liver in men occurred earlier (40-49 years) than in women (over 50 years) [35].

It was also reported that 5-20% of patients with NAFLD progressed to cirrhosis (non-alcoholic steatohepatitis; NASH) over a 10-year period [36]. Also in the prevalence of NASH in Japan, the peak for males was 25-34-year age group, while the peak for females was 55-74-year age group [37].

Although the sex or gender differences in the degree of fibrosis in patients with NAFLD were not identical, women tend to predominate among patients with severe fibrosis, as compared with those with mild fibrosis [38, 39]. In a cross-sectional study with Japanese 193 NASH patients, risk factors for advanced fibrosis according to the multivariate analysis were age and BMI in the younger group (<55 years), and the absence of hyperlipidemia in the older group (≥55 years) [37]. The prevalence of advanced fibrosis showed no gender differences in both the younger and the older groups [37].

In mice with steatohepatitis induced by methionine and choline-deficient diet, there were no sex differences in liver injury [40]. However, hepatic steatosis became evident in aromatase-deficient mice lacking intrinsic estrogen production, but substantially diminished in mice treated with 17-β-estradiol [41]. The role of estrogen in hepatic lipid metabolism and fibrosis remains to be further investigated.

5. AUTOIMMUNE LIVER DISEASES

It is well known that there are sex differences in the immune system. Females have higher immunoglobulin levels and mount stronger immune responses following immunization or infection than males [42-45]. *In vitro*, estrogen increased IgG and IgM production of peripheral blood mononuclear cells (PMBC) from both men and women [46, 47]. It has also been shown that estrogens increased and testosterone decreased autoantibody production of PMBC from patients with systemic lupus erythematosus [48, 49].

In addition, sex hormone levels in both humans and experimental models correlated with the activity of their cytokine-secreting cells. Serum dehydroepiandrosterone (DHEAS) level closely correlated with the activity of IFNγ-secreting cells in men and premenopausal women [50]. *In vitro*, DHEAS stimulated IFNγ production by murine lymphocyte [51], and promoted the production of IL-2, another type 1 cytokine [52]. The number of PBMC capable of secreting IL-4 was closely associated with serum estrogen level in women [50]. Estrogen addition increased the number of IL-6- and IL-10-secreting cells in the spleen of female mice [53]. Therefore, estrogen may activate B cell partially by stimulating type 2 cytokines (IL-4, IL-6 and IL-10).

These results suggest that estrogen or androgen may modulate the immune system, resulting in extended sex differences in autoimmune liver diseases.

6. AUTOIMMUNE HEPATITIS

Autoimmune hepatitis (AIH) occurs frequently in women aged between 10 and 30 years or during late middle age [54]. Women account for 70-90% of AIH patients [55, 56]. Miyake *et al.* reported that male patients with AIH showed a lower frequency of reproducibility in diagnosis with the revised scoring system proposed by the International Autoimmune Hepatitis Group [57], and a lower serum immunoglobulin G (IgG) level than female patients in Japan [58]. In addition, the frequency of normalization of the serum ALT level within 6 months after the beginning of corticosteroid treatment was significantly lower in men (73%) as compared with women (93%) [58]. On the other hand, there was no sex difference in age, form of clinical onset, frequency of symptomatic concurrent autoimmune diseases, and human leukocyte antigen DR (HLA DR) status [58]. In the UK, the frequencies of concurrent autoimmune diseases and HLA DR4 were significantly higher in women than in men, while there were no sex or gender differences in the serum IgG level and response to corticosteroid treatment [59]. These regional differences might arise from the fact that the clinical feature of AIH is different between patients with HLA DR3 and those with DR4 [60], and that most Japanese patients with AIH have HLA DR4 [61].

The severity of AIH was likely to decrease during pregnancy when estrogen was secreted at high levels, and acute exacerbation could occur after delivery [62]. In contrast, de novo presentation of AIH or its flaring in disease activity was also shown during pregnancy [63].

7. PRIMARY BILIARY CIRRHOSIS

Most patients with primary biliary cirrhosis (PBC) are female, usually 40-60 years of age [55]. Published data on the ratios of incidence in women to men ranged from 3:1 to 22:1 [64]. The complication of hepatocellular carcinoma (HCC) in patients with PBC was reported to be significantly greater in men than in women [65]. Age at the time of diagnosis, male sex, and history of blood transfusion were three independent factors of developing HCC in PBC patients who had negative markers for both HBV and HCV, and the combination of age, male sex and advanced-stage PBC was associated with patients' survival [66]. It was reported that concomitant autoimmune diseases, especially sicca syndrome, were less prevalent in men [65]. However, there was no serological difference between men and women [64].

8. PRIMARY SCLEROSING CHOLANGITIS (PSC)

In the Mayo Clinic study of 174 patients with primary sclerosing cholangitis (PSC), two-thirds were men and the mean age at the time of diagnosis was 39 years [67].

In an analysis of 388 Japanese patients with PSC,68 there was male predominance (59%) and two peaks in the age distribution, with a mean age of 47 years. The first peak was found in the group of PSC patients with inflammatory bowel diseases (IBD) who were mainly in their teens or twenties; the second peak was in the group of 50-60-year-olds, in which there were some patients with complications of autoimmune pancreatitis (AIP). The percentage of sex distribution did not differ among the three subgroups; PSC with IBD, PSC with AIP, and PSC without AIP.

9. HCC

Male predominance among patients with HCC is observed in high-risk as well as low-risk areas, regardless of ethnic and geographic diversities [69]. At present, the exact reason for such sex or gender differences is unclear. Heavy, long-term alcohol use, cigarette smoking and diabetes are known to be risk factors for HCC [70]. The sex or gender difference may be attributed to differences in exposure to these risk factors. However, among patients with cirrhotic NASH, whose ethanol intake was less than 100 g per week, the prevalence of HCC was higher in men (62%) compared with women (38%) [71].

In mouse model with HCC induced by diethylnitrosamine (DEN), serum IL-6 concentration and the incidence of HCC were higher in males compared with females [72]. The sex differences were abolished by ablation of IL-6, and estrogen inhibited secretion of IL-6 in males [72]. In chronic hepatitis C patients, the incidence rate of HCC increased in accordance with serum IL-6 level only in females, but there was no significant correlation between serum IL-6 level and estradiol level [73].

According to our investigations, the age at diagnosis of HCC was older in women (70 years) than in men (67 years), and the platelet count was significantly lower in women ($8.8 \pm 3.9 \times 10^4/mm^3$: mean $\pm$ SD) than in men ($11.3 \pm 4.5 \times 10^4/mm^3$) among 99 patients with positive HCV RNA (Nagoshi S, 2007, unpublished data). This finding suggests that women may develop HCC in more advanced stages of liver fibrosis than men. In Japan, there was no sex or gender difference in the incidence rate of having cirrhosis in patients with HCC, although women were diagnosed at significantly older age than men [74]. In contrast, Cong *et al.* showed that women with HCC were younger than men and that only 49% of women with HCC had cirrhosis in contrast to 68% among men in China [75]. Such discrepancies may be attributed to the differences in the prevalence of HBV and HCV infections. The positive rates of having HBsAg in patients with HCC were 11% in men and 7% in women in Japan [74], and 71% in men and 60% in women in China [75]

It has been reported that female patients with HCC showed better survival rates than male patients [74, 76, 77]. Some papers suggest that the better prognosis in female patients might relate to high incidence of tumor encapsulation and less invasive tumors [76], lower tumor recurrence rate [77], and the presence of lower numbers of androgen receptors in HCC.78 Interestingly the reason for the better prognosis in female patients with the same risk was reported to be ascribed to more frequent follow-up for the early diagnosis of HCC development than male patients [74]. Also, no significant sex or gender difference in the survival rate was reported in HCC patients [79].

10. CONCLUSION

Sex and gender specific medicine is an up-to-date issue to be solved from the standpoint of bio-sociology and bio-economics, including racial and geographic cultures.

The most important requirement for clinicians and medical scientists must be to establish the diagnosis, therapy, and prophylaxis based on the most advanced sex and gender specific medicine using recent scientific and medical tequniques towards extended quality of life and human happiness.

DISCLOSURE STATEMENT

Part of information included in this chapter has been previously published in *Hepatology Research* 38(3): 219-224, 2008.

REFERENCES

[1]   Blumberg BS, Sutnick AI, London WT, Melartin L. Sex distribution of Australia antigen. Arch Intern Med 1972; 130: 227-31.

[2]   Tanaka J, Kumagai J, Katayama K, *et al.* Sex- and age-specific carriers of hepatitis B and C viruses in Japan estimated by the prevalence in the 3 485 648 first-time blood donors during 1995-2000. Intervirology 2004; 47: 32-40.

[3]   Kashiwagi S, Hayashi J, Ikematsu H, *et al.* An epidemiologic study of hepatitis B virus in Okinawa and Kyushu, Japan. Am J Epidemiol 1983; 118: 787-94.

[4]   Furusyo N, Hayashi J, Sawayama Y, Kishihara Y, Kashiwagi S. Hepatitis B surface antigen disappearance and hepatitis B surface antigen subtype: a prospective, long-term, follow-up study of Japanese residents of Okinawa, Japan with chronic hepatitis B virus infection. Am J Trop Med Hyg 1999; 60: 616-22.

[5]   Verthelyi D. Sex hormones as immunomodulators in health and disease. Int Immunopharmacol 2001; 1: 983-93.

[6]   Sasaki T, Hattori T, Mayumi M. A large-scale survey on the prevalence of HBeAg and anti-HBe among asymptomatic carriers of HBV. Correlation with sex, age, HBsAg titre and s-GPT value. Vox Sang 1979; 37: 216-21.

[7]   Yuen MF, Yuan HJ, Hui CK, *et al.* A large population study of spontaneous HBeAg seroconversion and acute exacerbation of chronic hepatitis B infection: implications for antiviral therapy. Gut 2003; 52: 416-9.

[8]   Matsuura K, Tanaka Y, Hige S, *et al.* Distribution of hepatitis B virus genotypes among patients with chronic infection in Japan shifting toward an increase of genotype A. J Clin Microbiol 2009; 47: 1476-83.

[9]   Zacharakis G, Koskinas J, Kotsiou S, *et al.* Natural history of chronic hepatitis B virus infection in children of different ethnic origins: a cohort study with up to 12 years' follow-up in northern Greece. J Pediatr Gastroenterol Nutr 2007; 44: 84-91.

[10]   Chu CM, Liaw YF. Predictive factors for reactivation of hepatitis B following hepatitis B e antigen seroconversion in chronic hepatitis B. Gastroenterol 2007; 133: 1458-65.

[11]   Fattovich G, Brollo L, Giustina G, *et al.* Natural history and prognostic factors for chronic hepatitis type B. Gut 1991; 32: 294-8.

[12]   Bakr I, Rekacewicz C, El Hosseiny M, *et al.* Higher clearance of hepatitis C virus infection in females compared with males. Gut 2006; 55: 1183-7.

[13]   Yazdanpanah Y, De Carli G, Migueres B, *et al.* Risk factors for hepatitis C virus transmission to health care workers after occupational exposure: a European case-control study. Clin Infect Dis 2005; 41: 1423-30.

[14]   Toyoda H, Kumada T, Kiriyama S, *et al.* Influence of age, sex, and degree of liver fibrosis on the association between serum alanine aminotransferase levels and liver inflammation in patients with chronic hepatitis C. Dig Dis Sci 2004; 49: 295-9.

[15]   Mochida S, Hashimoto M, Matsui A, *et al.* genetic polymorphism in promoter region of osteopontin gene may be a marker reflecting hepatitis activity in chronic hepatitis C patients. Biochem Biophys Res Com 2004; 313: 1079-85.

[16]   Rodriguez-Torres M, Rios-Bedoya CF, Rodriguez-Orengo J, *et al.* Progression to cirrhosis in Latinos with chronic hepatitis C: differences in Puerto Ricans with and without human immunodeficiency virus coinfection and along gender. J Clin Gastroenterol 2006; 40: 358-66.

[17]   Wright M, Goldin R, Fabre A, *et al.* Measurement and determinants of the natural history of liver fibrosis in hepatitis C virus infection: a cross sectional and longitudinal study. Gut 2003; 52: 574-9.

[18]   Poynard T, Mathurin P, Lai CL, *et al.* A comparison of fibrosis progression in chronic liver diseases. J Hepatol 2003; 38: 257-65.

[19]   Poynard T, Ratziu V, Charlotte F, *et al.* Rates and risk factors of liver fibrosis progression in patients with chronic hepatitis C. J Hepatol 2001; 34: 730-9.

[20]   Boccato S, Pistis R, Noventa F, *et al.* Fibrosis progression in initially mild chronic hepatitis C. J Viral Hepat 2006; 13: 297-302.

[21]   Minola E, Prati D, Suter F, *et al.* Age at infection affects the long-term outcome of transfusion-associated chronic hepatitis C. Blood 2002; 99: 4588-91.

[22]   Murakami C, Hino K, Korenaga M, *et al.* Factors predicting progression to cirrhosis and hepatocellular carcinoma in patients with transfusion-associated hepatitis C virus infection. J Clin Gastroenterol 1999; 28: 148-52.

[23]   Sezaki H, Suzuki F, Akuta N, *et al.* Influence of gender to efficacy of interferon/ribavirin combination therapy in chronic hepatitis C patients in Japan. Kanzo 2007; 48: 296-8.

[24]   Conjeevaram HS, Fried MW, Jeffers LJ, *et al.* Peginterferon and ribavirin treatment in African American and Caucasian American patients with hepatitis C genotype 1. Gastroenterology 2006; 131: 470-7.

[25]   Tanaka Y, Nishida N, Sugiyama M, *et al.* Genome-wide association of IL28B with response to pegylated interferon-a and ribavirin therapy for chronic hepatitis C. Nat med 2009; 41: 1105-9.

[26]   Ge D Fellay J, Thompson AJ, Simon JS, *et al.* Genetic variation in IL28B predicts hepatitis C treatment-induced viral clearance. Nature 2009; 461: 399-401.

[27]   Becker U, Deis A, Sørensen TI *et al.* Prediction of risk of liver disease by alcohol intake, sex, and age: a prospective population study. Hepatology 1996; 23: 1025-9.

[28]   Frezza M, di Padova C, Pozzato G, *et al.* High blood alcohol levels in women. The role of decreased gastric alcohol dehydrogenase activity and first-pass metabolism. N Engl J Med 1990; 322: 95-9.

[29]   Baraona E, Abittan CS, Dohmen K, *et al.* Gender differences in pharmacokinetics of alcohol. Alcohol Clin Exp Res 2001; 25: 502-7.

[30]   Thurman RG. Sex-related liver injury due to alcohol involves activation of Kupffer cells by endotoxin. Can J Gastroenterol 2000; 14 Suppl D: 129D-135D.

[31]   Järveläinen HA, Lukkari TA, Heinaro S, *et al.* The antiestrogen toremifene protects against alcoholic liver injury in female rats. J Hepatol 2001; 35: 46-52.

[32]   Niemelä O, Parkkila S, Pasanen M, *et al.* Induction of cytochrome P450 enzymes and generation of protein-aldehyde adducts are associated with sex-dependent sensitivity to alcohol-induced liver disease in micropigs. Hepatology 1999; 30: 1011-7.

[33]   Chitturi S, Farrell GC, Hashimoto E, et al; the Asia-Pacific Working Party on NAFLD. Non-alcoholic fatty liver disease in the Asia-Pacific region: definitions and overview of proposed guidelines. J Gastroenterol Hepatol 2007; 22: 778-87.

[34]   Kojima S, Watanabe N, Numata M, *et al.* Increase in the prevalence of fatty liver in Japan over the past 12 years: analysis of clinical background. J Gastroenterol 2003; 38: 954-61.

[35]   Fan JG, Zhu J, Li XJ, *et al.* Prevalence of and risk factors for fatty liver in a general population of Shanghai, China. J Hepatol 2005; 43: 508-14.

[36]   Farrell GC, Larter CZ. Nonalcoholic fatty liver disease: from steatosis to cirrhosis. Hepatology 2006; 43: S99-S112.

[37]   Yatsuji S, Hashimoto E, Tobari M, *et al.* Influence of age and gender in Japanese patients with non-alcoholic steatohepatitis. Hepatol Res 2007; 37: 1034-43.

[38] Fan JG, Saibara T, Chitturi S, et al; the Asia-Pacific Working Party for NAFLD. What are the risk factors and settings for non-alcoholic fatty liver disease in Asia-Pacific? J Gastroenterol Hepatol 2007; 22: 794-800.

[39] Angulo P, Keach JC, Batts KP, Lindor KD. Independent predictors of liver fibrosis in patients with nonalcoholic steatohepatitis. Hepatology 1999; 30: 1356-62.

[40] Kashireddy PR, Rao MS. Sex differences in choline-deficient diet-induced steatohepatitis in mice. Exp Biol Med 2004; 229: 158-62.

[41] Nemoto Y, Toda K, Ono M, *et al*. Altered expression of fatty acid-metabolizing enzymes in aromatase-deficient mice. J Clin Invest 2000; 105: 1819-25.

[42] Schuurs AHWM, Verheul HAM. Effects of gender and sex hormones on the immune response. Steroid Biochem 1990; 35: 157-72.

[43] Grossman CJ. Interactions between gonadal steroids and the immune system. Science 1985; 227: 257-61.

[44] Ansar Ahmed S, Penhale WP, Talal N. Sex hormones, immune responses and autoimmune diseases: mechanisms of sex hormone action. Am J Pathol 1985; 121: 531-51.

[45] Da Silva JAP. Sex hormones, glucocorticoids and autoimmunity: facts and hypotheses. Ann Rheum Dis 1995; 54: 6-16.

[46] Kanda N, Tamaki K. Estrogen enhances immunoglobulin production by human PBMCs. J Allergy Clin Immunol 1999; 103: 282

[47] Weetman, AP, McGregor AM, Smith BR, Hall R. Sex hormones enhance immunoglobulin synthesis by human peripheral blood lymphocytes. Immunol Lett 1981; 3: 343.

[48] Kanda N, Tsuchida T, Tamaki K. Estrogen enhancement of anti-double-stranded DNA antibody and immunoglobulin G production in peripheral blood mononuclear cells from patients with systemic lupus erythematosus. Arthritis Rheum 1999; 42: 328-37.

[49] Kanda N, Tsuchida T, Tamaki K. Testosterone suppresses anti-DNA antibody production in peripheral blood mononuclear cells from patients with systemic lupus erythmatosus. Arthritis Rheum 1997; 40: 1703-11.

[50] Verthelyi D, Klinman DM. Sex hormone levels correlate with the activity of cytokine-secreting cells *in vivo*. Immunology 2000; 10: 384-90.

[51] Kim HR, Ryu SY, Kim HS, *et al*. Administration of dehydroepiandrosterone reverses the immune suppression induced by high doses of antigen in mice. Immunol Invest 1995; 24: 83-93.

[52] Daynes RA, Dudley DJ, Araneo BA. Regulation of murine lymphokine production *in vivo*: II. Dehydroepiandrosteron is a natural enhancer of interleukin 2 synthesis by helper T cells. Eur J Immunol 1990; 20: 793-802.

[53] Verthelyi D. Sex hormones as immunomodulators in health and disease. Intern Immunopharm 2001; 1: 983-993.

[54] Schiff ER, Sorrell MF, Maddrey WC. Schiff's Disease of the Liver. Philadelphia, PA: Lippincott Williams & Wilkins, 2006.

[55] Sherlock S, Dooley J. Diseases of the Liver and Biliary System. Oxford: Blackwell Science, 2002.

[56] Zakim D, Boyer TD. Zakim and Boyer's Hepatology a Textbook of Liver Disease. Philadelphia, PA: W.B. Saunders 2006.

[57] Alvarez F, Berg PA, Bianchi FB, *et al*. International Autoimmune Hepatitis Group Report: review of criteria for diagnosis of autoimmune hepatitis. J Hepatol 1999; 31: 929-38.

[58] Miyake Y, Iwasaki Y, Sakaguchi K, Shiratori Y. Clinical features of Japanese male patients with type 1 autoimmune hepatitis. Aliment Pharmacol Ther 2006; 24: 519-23.

[59] Czaja AJ, Donaldson PT. Gender effects and synergisms with histocompatibility leukocyte antigens in type 1 autoimmune hepatitis. Am J Gastroenterol 2002; 97: 2051-7.

[60] Czaja AJ, Freese DK. American association for the study of liver disease. Diagnosis and treatment of autoimmune hepatitis. Hepatology 2002; 36: 479-97.

[61] Toda G, Zeniya M, Watanabe F, *et al*. Present status of autoimmune hepatitis in Japan-correlating the characteristics with international criteria in an area with a high rate of HCV infection. Japanese National Study Group of Autoimmune Hepatitis. J Hepatol 1997; 26: 1207-12.

[62] Buchel E, Van Steenbergen W, Nevens F, Fevery J. Improvement of autoimmune hepatitis during pregnancy followed by flare-up after delivery. Am J Gastroenterol 2002; 97: 3160-5.

[63] Heneghan MA, Norris SM, O'Grady JG, *et al*. Management and outcome of pregnancy in autoimmune hepatitis. Gut 2001; 48: 97-102.

[64] Nalbandian G, Van de Water J, Gish R, *et al*. Is there a serological difference between men and women with primary biliary cirrhosis? Am J Gastroenterol 1999; 94: 2482-6.

[65]   Lucey MR, Neuberger JM, Williams R. Primary biliary cirrhosis in men. Gut 1986; 27: 1373-6.

[66]   Shibuya A, Tanaka K, Miyakawa H, *et al.* Hepatocellular carcinoma and survival in patients with primary biliary cirrhosis. Hepatology 2002; 35: 1172-8.

[67]   Wiesner RH, Grambsch PM, Dickson ER, *et al.* Primary sclerosing cholangitis: natural history, prognostic factors and survival analysis. Hepatology 1989; 10: 430-6.

[68]   Takikawa H, Takamori Y, Tanaka A, *et al.* Analysis of 388 cases of primary sclerosing cholangitis in Japan; Presence of a subgroup without pancreatic involvement in older patients. Hepatol Res 2004; 29: 153-9.

[69]   El-Serag HB. Hepatocellular carcinoma: an epidemiologic view. J Clin Gastroentero 2002; 35: S72-8.

[70]   Yu MC, Yuan JM. Environmental factors and risk for hepatocellular carcinoma. Gastroenterol 2004; 127 (5 Suppl 1): S72-8.

[71]   Hashimoto E, Yatsuji S, Tobari M, *et al.* Hepatocellular carcinoma in patients with nonalcoholic steatohepatitis. J Gastroenterol 2009; 44 Suppl 19: 89-95.

[72]   Naugler WE, Sakurai T, Kim S, *et al.* Gender disparity in liver cancer due to sex differences in MyD88-dependent IL-6 production. Science 2007; 317: 121-4.

[73]   Nakagawa H, Maeda S, Yoshida H, *et al.* Serum IL-6 levels and the risk for hepatocarcinogenesis in chronic hepatitis C patients: an analysis based on gender differences. Int J Cancer 2009; 125: 2264-9.

[74]   Dohmen K, Shigematsu H, Irie K, Ishibashi H. Longer survival in female than male with hepatocellular carcinoma. J Gastroenterol Hepatol 2003; 18: 267-72.

[75]   Cong WM, Wu MC, Zhang XH, *et al.* Primary hepatocellular carcinoma in women of mainland China. A clinicopathologic analysis of 104 patients. Cancer 1993; 71: 2941-5.

[76]   Ng IO, Ng MM, Lai EC, Fan ST. Better survival in female patients with hepatocellular carcinoma. Possible causes from a pathologic approach. Cancer 1995; 75: 18-22.

[77]   Ng IO, Ng M, Fan ST. Better survival in women with resected hepatocellular carcinoma is not related to tumor proliferation or expression of hormone receptors. Am J Gastroenterol 1997; 92: 1355-8.

[78]   Nagasue N, Kohno H, Chang YC, *et al.* Androgen and estrogen receptors in hepatocellular carcinoma and the surrounding liver in women. Cancer 1989; 63: 112-6.

[79]   El-Serag HB, Mason AC, Key C. Trends in survival of patients with hepatocellular carcinoma between 1977 and 1996 in the United States. Hepatology 2001; 33: 62-5.

Index

www.ingramcontent.com/pod-product-compliance
Lightning Source LLC
Chambersburg PA
CBHW041718210326
41598CB00007B/694